THE SMART GUIDE TO

Nutrition

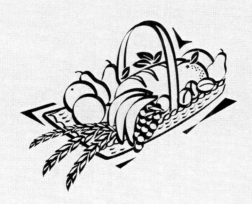

BY ANNE MACZULAK

SECOND EDITION

The Smart Guide To Nutrition - Second Edition

Published by

Smart Guide Publications, Inc.
2517 Deer Chase Drive
Norman, OK 73071
www.smartguidepublications.com

For information, address: Smart Guide Publications, Inc. 2517 Deer Creek Drive, Norman, OK 73071

SMART GUIDE and Design are registered trademarks licensed to Smart Guide Publications, Inc.

International Standard Book Number: 9781937636753

Library of Congress Catalog Card Number:
11 12 13 14 15   10 9 8 7 6 5 4 3 2 1

Printed in the United States of America

Cover design: Lorna Llewellyn
Copy Editor: Ruth Strother
Back cover design: Joel Friedlander, Eric Gelb, Deon Seifert
Back cover copy: Eric Gelb, Deon Seifert
Illustrations: James Balkovek
Production: Zoë Lonergan
Indexer: Cory Emberson
V.P./Business Manager: Cathy Barker

ACKNOWLEDGMENTS

I wish to give special thanks to the teachers and advisors who guided my training in animal nutrition at the Ohio State University and the University of Kentucky. I thank Burk Dehority, James Boling, and William Tyznik for guidance and encouragement. I also wish to thank the Smart Guide series publisher and copy ediotr Ruth Strother for their sound editorial advice and illustrator James Balkovek. Much gratitude goes to my agent Jodie Rhodes for her unending support.

Sincere thanks go to my father, Leon Maczulak, for his support throughout my career.

Finally, I owe a special acknowledgment to my friend Moose who played a key and unforgettable part in my nutrition studies in Kentucky.

TABLE OF CONTENTS

18 Essential Minerals: The Trace Elements

INTRODUCTION

Nutrition is a science in which you conduct experiments every day. When you select fruit over candy, milk over beer, or granola instead of a hot dog, you affect your body's metabolism. In this book you will learn the meaning of *metabolism* and see how nutrition connects with a variety of other scientific fields. Where else could you pick up a book seeking to learn about proteins and vitamins and at the same time enrich your knowledge of chemistry, medicine, agriculture, biochemistry, and microbiology?

This Smart Guide explains nutrition from the ground up, sometimes literally when you consider the plant life that brings nutrients to all other living things. By starting with the basics of cell chemistry, you see where the nutrients from food actually go after you eat a meal.

The Smart Guide to Nutrition covers individual nutrient classes and today's popular nutrients that come not in food but in a bottle. Do multivitamins work? Is it safe to take zinc supplements? Are you getting enough antioxidants? This book gives you a sound background in nutrition so that you can answer these questions intelligently and based on facts. It's time to separate the scientific facts from myth, and few scientific subjects carry more myths than nutrition!

Do you think you are what you eat? This book shows how we grow, reproduce, and age depending on our food choices. But at the end of the day, all our bodies are more similar than they are different as far as how we digest foods, absorb nutrients, transport those nutrients to cells, and use them for energy.

Energy. It is the theme of all the chapters in this Smart Guide book . You will learn here how all your dietary choices ultimately go toward providing you with either enough energy to enjoy your life, or not enough to get through a day without feeling tired.

This book covers the essential nutrient groups, the basic food groups, and the common mistakes people make when selecting foods. Some of these mistakes can seriously harm your health, so nutrition is an important subject to learn even at a young age, but certainly as an adult and as you age. You will be introduced to proteins, carbohydrates, fats, vitamins, minerals, and even water; and you'll learn what they do in your body and how you can help them work even better.

You will also learn something about the various diets that are part of nutrition the world over. There exists no single correct path to good nutrition; you can achieve good nutrition a number of different ways. And that is what makes nutrition fun!

The *Smart Guide to Nutrition* is a handy resource for the basics of nutrition from simple molecules to the whole body.

PART ONE

Nutrition and Digestion

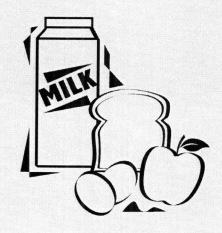

CHAPTER 1

 # The Basics of Nutrition

In This Chapter

➤ Learning what is nutrition and what makes food

➤ Several ways to know your body's composition

➤ Energy sources and the types of food energy

In this chapter you will begin to learn what makes good nutrition. First of all, what is nutrition? How is nutrition different from diet, and how does the word *diet* differ from *dieting*?

This chapter also begins a theme you'll discover throughout this book, that is, how to distinguish good nutrition choices from bad nutrition choices. This is a very important subject because few areas of science receive as much misinformation and downright dangerous myths as nutrition.

I can save you some time. For seeking sound advice on nutrition, avoid friends who run from one popular fad to the next, be wary of the advice and supplements promoted by athletic clubs and gyms, and watch out for eye-catching magazine articles on cure-all nutrients. Do you really think there is a secret nutrient that will recharge your sex life? Can a soft drink give you an extra five hours of power-packed energy? Is that stuff in the refrigerated section really brain food?

Nutrition is a science, but unlike nuclear physics or molecular biology, it is a science for the masses. We make our own nutrition decisions every day. To make the best decisions possible, you should seek out the best resources for topics in nutrition. This means going to professionals for advice, mainly physicians, nutritionists, and registered dieticians. When you look for information on the Internet, avoid magazine-style articles or any chat or blog that lacks references or resources.

Where should a person go to seek the right information on nutrition? Start with this book! To add to your knowledge on any subject covered in these pages, go to the websites of the Food and Drug Administration (FDA), www.fda.gov; the U.S. Department of Agriculture (USDA), www.usda.gov; universities such as the Harvard School of Public Health, www. hsph.harvard.edu; and professional organizations such as the American Society for Nutrition, www.nutrition.org. Most of these organizations have ways for you to contact a scientist by e-mail or phone to receive answers to a specific nutrition question.

Let's begin by making sure you are holding the correct book. Do you know what nutrition is?

What Is Nutrition?

Nutrition is a science focused on the ways your body uses substances in food to maintain life. These vital substances contained in food are called *nutrients*.

Scientists are fond of saying that people eat food, not nutrients. This is true not only for humans but for every other animal. Only plants and microbes ingest mainly nutrients rather than food.

Good nutrition involves making choices in the types and amounts of foods you eat daily to promote good health. Poor nutrition involves the opposite of all those decisions!

The Difference between Good and Poor Nutrition

It seems easy. Take a piece of paper and write down all the factors that you think go into making up good nutrition. You will probably come up with things like eating three square meals a day, consuming plenty of fresh fruits and vegetables, and avoiding overeating. But opinions about nutrition vary widely these days. It may not be easy to tell good from bad nutritional decisions.

Does the following list seem like good nutrition or poor nutrition?

> ➤ To lose weight, a woman drastically reduces her daily food intake until she feels weak and lightheaded.

> ➤ To combat a stressful work situation, a man gorges each night on nachos, pizza, and beer.

> ➤ To make the team, one teenager has only high-energy drinks for breakfast, and another teenager bulks up on a high-protein diet and steroids.

➤ Following the lead of a movie star, a college student turns to a vegan diet espoused by a popular fashion magazine.

➤ To combat cancer, a salesperson eats a macrobiotic diet described by a physician on a morning TV news show.

➤ To support her new exercise program, a therapist takes the advice of her trainer and eliminates all carbohydrates from her diet.

Are these examples of good decisions or poor decisions? The first three seem like pretty lousy decisions for maintaining health, and they are truly dangerous approaches to nutrition. The last three seem like poor nutrition decisions also, but in fact may not be. Perhaps the vegan diet printed in the fashion magazine contains sound nutritional advice from a trained professional. Perhaps the trainer at the gym is also a nutritionist who will guide his client to a healthy low-carbohydrate diet. What about the physician on the morning TV show? Is this a physician who is respected in the field of nutrition and has done years of research on the connection between cancer and diet? Or is this physician a best-selling author who just came out with a new paperback titled *The Kick-Cancer Diet*?

Because we cannot always be certain of the quality of nutrition advice we get from magazines, TV, radio, and many online sources, we must arm ourselves with knowledge. By understanding how the body gets nutrients from food, and what the body does with those nutrients, you can make better nutrition choices for yourself and for your family.

We control our own nutrition by the type of diet we consume. In this book, diet is the main types of nutrient sources you eat in a given time period. For example, diets can be vegetarian, non-vegetarian, high-fiber, and so forth. The term *dieting* refers to the consumption of a certain diet for a specific purpose, such as weight loss.

Once you learn the nuts and bolts of nutrition, you can stop worrying

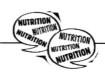

Nutrition Vocabulary

Let's learn about food processing. All food receives some processing unless you go out to your garden and chomp on lettuce leaves like a rabbit. Minimal processing involves only picking a raw vegetable or fruit and perhaps rinsing it with water. Many foods today receive much more extensive processing. For raw salad vegetables this may include the washing, trimming, and packaging after harvest. Canned and frozen foods receive the most processing. Some of the things they might be subjected to are cooking, mixing, preservatives, flavor and color enhancers, wrapping, vacuum packing, freezing, or irradiating. As a general rule, each step in the processing scheme can destroy a portion of the nutrients that were in the fresh food before harvesting.

about nutrients, calories, carbs, and any other topic of the month in nutrition, and simply pick the best foods in building a diet to maintain good health.

What Makes Food?

Food is the body's source of all the nutrients it needs to stay alive. This means that a can of Spaghetti-O's is food just as much as a freshly picked stalk of broccoli is food. Some people might argue that a can of processed food can hardly be called food at all. But if the stuff inside the container can be digested by a person and supply nutrients, it is a food.

Almost all mammals need some variety in the foods they eat. In other words, there is no single perfect food that supplies all the nutrients a body needs. Thus, we know foods as different groups: vegetables, meat, dairy products, grains, and so on. The trick to good nutrition is to accomplish three things:

1. Select a variety of foods that complement each other in the variety and amount of nutrients they supply.

2. Avoid placing too much emphasis on any one food causing you to exclude other food groups, such as eating a pound of carrots every day.

3. Select foods that give you the energy needed for your particular lifestyle and do not lead to dramatic weight loss or weight gain.

The last principle of good nutrition mentioned above applies to people who are within a weight range ideal for their height, sex, and age. Unfortunately, lots of people are not within their ideal weight range or have health issues related to their nutrition. They may make food decisions for the wrong reasons. It is important to remember what food is not:

> ➤ Food is not a drug. This means food is not intended as a treatment for disease.

> ➤ Food is not an aphrodisiac. Food is not a substance intended to arouse sexual desire.

> ➤ Food is not currency. Food should not be used to bribe someone, like a child, into doing something you wish them to do. In war-torn regions of the world, food should not be withheld from people to make them agree with political objectives.

> ➤ Food is not punishment. Food should not be forced on anyone as a penalty for certain behavior, in hazing, in reality TV shows, or as a practical joke.

In this book, I hope to disconnect the emotions that go with certain foods or eating behaviors. I hope to help you learn exactly what food is: a source of chemicals that go into building your body's bones and muscles, nerves and blood, and every other type of tissue that makes up the body.

Your Body's Chemical Composition

The easiest way to take the emotion out of food—and maybe some of the romance, too—is to look at your body's composition. The chemicals that make up the human body are, after all, supplied directly by your nutrition.

The body can be broken down into components in several different ways. The easiest breakdown is according to water and non-water components. By this breakdown, a lean person contains about 60 percent water and 40 percent non-water components. Of the 40 percent non-water components, the body is made of fat (17 percent), protein (17 percent), and bone (6 percent).

The amount of fat in the body, called body fat, can be measured to determine if a person is within their ideal weight range, underweight, overweight, or obese. This measurement is called a body mass index (BMI) and is covered in more detail later in this book.

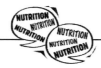

Nutrition Vocabulary

Think of the terms *underweight*, *lean*, *overweight*, and *obese*. These words appear in many discussions of nutrition. No single ideal body weight exists for humans. Scientists prefer to describe optimal weight in a range. Anyone within their optimal weight range for their height, sex, and age can be called lean. A person whose weight falls outside the lowest end of the ideal range is underweight. A person who is outside the highest end of the ideal range is overweight. An overweight person who exceeds a certain percentage of body fat is said to be obese.

Water consists only of hydrogen and oxygen. Chemically, you know water as H_2O. But fat, protein, and bone carry many other chemical elements. We can break down the body into its chemical composition based on body weight this way:

➤ Oxygen: 61–65 percent

➤ Carbon: 18.5–23.0 percent

➤ Hydrogen: 9.5–10.0 percent

➤ Nitrogen: 2.6–3.3 percent

➤ Calcium: 1.4–1.5 percent

➤ Phosphorus: 0.8–1.0 percent

➤ Potassium: about 0.4 percent

➤ Sulfur: about 0.3 percent

➤ Sodium: about 0.2 percent

➤ Chlorine: about 0.2 percent

➤ Magnesium: about 0.1 percent

➤ All other body elements make up the remaining 5 percent or less.

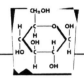

The Chemistry of Nutrition

The body is made of chemicals called elements. An element is a substance that cannot be broken down into any other substance. Thus, the element carbon contains only carbon atoms. Similarly, oxygen gas, which tends to be made of two oxygen atoms (O_2), when broken down yields only free oxygen atoms. Compare that to water, which can be broken down chemically into hydrogen and oxygen.

By the way, an atom is the smallest unit of matter. All the elements on Earth are composed of atoms.

But, What Am I?

Studying the chemical composition of the body gives you some clues as to why we need certain nutrients, such as calcium, but it still tells us little about what makes us human. All of the chemicals we call nutrients arrange themselves in the body to make proteins, fat, muscle, blood, etc. Therefore, your body composition can be described based by the way elements are arranged. Chemists call these arrangements molecules. The molecular makeup of the body's mass in percentage of body weight is:

➤ Water: 60 percent

➤ Fat: about 17 percent

➤ Protein: 14–17 percent

➤ Minerals, such as calcium and iron: 5.3 percent

➤ Lipids, fatlike substances: 2.1 percent

➤ Carbohydrates: 0.6 percent

Still not very helpful, is it? How about if I further arrange these molecules into categories that make a human body walk, talk, and live:

➤ Muscle: 40 percent

➤ Adipose tissue (the storage form of fat): 21.4 percent

➤ Blood: 7.9 percent

➤ Bone: 7.1 percent

➤ Skin: 3.7 percent

➤ Liver: 2.6 percent

➤ All other tissues: 17.3 percent

Now this is starting to look like a human! All these different types of tissues operate together to keep you alive. The chemical activities inside the cells that make up these tissues is called metabolism, and the whole purpose of nutrition is to keep your body metabolism running.

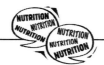

Nutrition Vocabulary

Just as an atom is the smallest unit in chemistry, a cell is the smallest unit that makes up a living organism. All plant and animal bodies are composed of cells. Microbes are single cells, but they are still cells. Only cells have a mechanism for bringing nutrients inside them and reproducing on their own.

The Meaning of Metabolism

Metabolism is the sum total of all chemical reactions in your body. This includes reactions that break down stored substances for energy. It also includes reactions that build large chemicals out of small ones to store energy to make new cells. Nutritionists call this building process building body mass.

Metabolism is the machinery that makes a body run. Plants have metabolism, animals have metabolism, and microbes all have diverse types of metabolism. Plant metabolism revolves around photosynthesis, the ability to convert the Sun's energy along with carbon dioxide into sugar. Microbes use a variety of metabolisms depending on where they live. Most animals have similar metabolism based on breathing in oxygen, using carbon compounds for building body mass, and exhaling carbon dioxide and other wastes.

The following are examples of activities that are part of your body metabolism:

➤ Digesting a cupcake

➤ Using the cupcake's sugars for energy

➤ Depositing the cupcake's fat (the icing!) in adipose tissue

➤ Burning some of the fats in adipose tissue when you decide to take a run around the block (guilt from eating the cupcake, perhaps?)

➤ Eliminating the waste products of those fat-burning reactions by way of the kidneys, skin, and lungs

All the nutrients you take in have the sole purpose of maintaining your metabolism. And the purpose of metabolism is to give you energy.

Energy

The body needs energy to operate just like a car needs energy to roll down the highway. You give your car energy in the form of a chemical: gasoline. The car's engine combusts the gasoline and converts the chemical energy into mechanical energy. This mechanical energy runs the car's systems when idling and also powers its motion.

Your body's gasoline is food. Food powers body metabolism. Like a car running because of its combustion engine, a body runs because of respiration. Respiration is the first step in converting the chemical energy stored in foods to other forms of energy, just like the engine converts gasoline's chemical energy into other forms of energy.

The combustion analogy actually works as well in nutrition as it does in the automotive world. Scientists determine the energy content of foods by putting the food in a contraption called a bomb calorimeter, and then like a bomb they combust the food. The heat given off by the explosion tells them the energy content of the food.

Where We Get Our Energy

Eating is all about giving your body's cells the energy they need to run chemical reactions. We harvest that energy from the foods we eat. Plants convert the Sun's energy directly into a usable form for us, mainly as carbohydrates and proteins.

Meat-producing animals take an extra step to deliver the Sun's energy to us. Cattle, for instance, graze on grasses that have captured solar energy and converted it to chemical energy. The cattle then convert the energy in the grass into another form of chemical energy stored in their tissues, mainly muscle and fat. So humans indirectly get the Sun's energy when we eat meat.

All of our food thus represents some sort of conversion of the Sun's energy (solar energy) into chemical energy the body can use.

Types of Food Energy

Animals never get all the energy out of food that food contains. The total quantity of energy in any food is its gross energy; that is, the energy scientists measure in a bomb calorimeter.

When we eat a meal, we digest a portion of the meal and a portion goes undigested and leaves the body as feces. The portion of gross energy that the body absorbs is called digestible energy.

Because of some inefficiencies in the body, not all digestible energy gets used. Some substances circulate through the bloodstream without being taken up by cells. The kidneys then remove these substances from the blood and excrete them in urine. Only the food energy that is actually used by cells is useful in metabolism. It is called metabolizable energy.

The metabolizable energy value of a food has a great impact on body maintenance, reproduction, and growth.

CHAPTER 2

Metabolism Made Easy

In This Chapter

➤ The meaning of metabolism and its two main components

➤ Examples of anabolism and catabolism

➤ The chemical reactions of your body

➤ How respiration works and why it's important

In this chapter you explore body metabolism in detail. Since the whole point of nutrition is to make your metabolism go, you can hardly claim to understand nutrition without knowing how your body keeps humming along.

Metabolism can be dissected into a simple equation:

$$\text{Food In} + \text{Wastes Out} = \text{Metabolism}$$

The food that goes into the body must first be digested into smaller components. For example, a steak and potato meal gets digested into meat proteins and the carbohydrates from the mashed potatoes. These products of digestion inside your digestive tract give you the nutrients you need. Nutrients must then be absorbed from the gut before entering the bloodstream. Finally, cells must absorb the nutrients from the blood before they can be used for metabolism.

Nutrition begins the instant you put a food into your mouth. It ends when you excrete wastes. These wastes leave the body by several routes:

➤ Solid, undigestible food leaves as feces from the digestive tract.

➤ Some metabolizable wastes leave the body in bile excreted by the liver and put into the digestive track via the gall bladder. Other metabolizable wastes exit the body in urine made by the kidneys and via the bladder.

➤ Excretions exit the body in sweat through the skin.

➤ Carbon dioxide exits the body via the lungs.

The events inside your body related to metabolizable nutrients determine your health. Metabolism has certain steadfast needs. Consider this scenario:

Think of yourself as a being that requires only ten nutrients to live. You eat a diet that gives you a rich supply of nutrients one through nine, but your diet totally lacks nutrient ten. Because your cells have an absolute requirement for all ten nutrients, they cannot run their metabolism because one nutrient is missing.

This is a critical point in the understanding of nutrition: only a balanced diet supports a body's metabolism. A balanced diet in appropriate relative amounts supplies all the nutrients to do two things:

1. Support metabolism

2. Nourish the body without the nutrients interfering with each other

Picture cells in a healthy, well-nourished person with a balanced diet compared to cells in a malnourished body. Healthy cell Hygeia (named for the Greek goddess of health) says, "Oh goody, here comes some blood. Let's see, I'll take calcium, phosphorus, these amino acids, some fats, and, oh yes, some of this nice sugar glucose. I'm all set for today!" Meanwhile, malnourished cell Limos (the Greek god of famine) has his own shopping list, but the blood does not meet his needs. He complains, "I need calcium, sulfur, phosphorus, magnesium, glucose, and about ten amino acids. But darn! All I'm getting is a ton of phosphorus and glucose and none of the other things I need. I'm starving!"

You simply cannot make up for the lack of one nutrient by taking in more of the other nutrients. Metabolism contains several interconnected pieces that work together only if they all get a steady input of the nutrients they must have.

Building Up and Breaking Down

At this moment, your cells are conducting a feverish series of steps that involves:

1. Absorbing nutrients needed to generate energy

2. Stocking away extra nutrients

3. Maybe breaking down a few stored substances to make up for any missing nutrients in the blood.

In other words, you can get away with missing a meal from time to time, or opting for a box of those little chocolate doughnuts instead of chicken salad because your cells make up the difference by taking some of the nutrients stored in your body. But this lasts for just a short time. Sooner, rather than later, you must return to a balanced diet to stay in good health.

The building up of substances in your body is called anabolism. Examples of anabolic processes are:

➤ Building bone to strengthen your skeleton

➤ Adding adipose tissue to your waistline or thighs

➤ Increasing muscle mass by weightlifting

➤ Storing extra carbon in your liver for when it is needed later

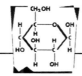

The Chemistry of Nutrition

Carbon makes up only 0.09 percent of Earth's crust but all life revolves around this single element. Any compound built on carbon is called an organic compound. More than 5 million organic compounds exist on Earth. These include the materials that make up coal, petroleum, industrial solvents such as benzene, and the foods that go into your body. Your body needs carbon almost everywhere. It goes into carbohydrates (the reason they are called *carbo-*), proteins, fats, and your genetic material, called nucleic acids. The metabolic process concerns moving carbon into and out of these substances for making new cells and generating energy.

Catabolism is the breakdown of substances in the body so cells can get the energy and nutrients they need to keep their metabolism running. Examples of catabolic processes are:

➤ Burning fat during an aerobics class

➤ Drawing on carbohydrates stored in the liver while running a marathon

➤ Losing muscle mass due to protein breakdown during a prolonged fast

➤ Feeding carbon from fats and blood sugar into energy-generating reactions while taking the SAT exam

The reactions of anabolism and catabolism involve mainly the carbon compounds we know as carbohydrates as well as fats and proteins. Vitamins and minerals play an auxiliary role in the buildup and breakdown reactions of metabolism.

One more thing to remember about anabolism and catabolism is that anabolism uses energy and catabolism releases energy. Therefore, to perform an anabolic activity like building up your muscles, you need to take in higher amounts of energy and nutrients, that is, you need to eat more food. When your body breaks down stored substances during catabolism to generate energy, you don't need to eat more. Instead of taking in extra food during catabolism, your body releases some extra energy in the form of heat.

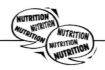

Nutrition Vocabulary

A carbohydrate is any carbon-containing compound assembled according to a generic chemical formula. For example, the sugar glucose is a carbohydrate containing six carbon atoms, twelve hydrogen atoms, and six oxygen atoms. Chemists put this formula into shorthand as $C_6H_{12}O_6$. Because it contains six carbons, chemists classify glucose as a hexose. Multiples of glucose exist in nature from two glucoses linked together to several dozen. These are all carbohydrates.

Some carbohydrates begin with a five-carbon, rather than a six-carbon base unit. These are collectively called pentoses and are represented by the formula $C_5H_{10}O_5$.

By now, you may have deduced that the generic chemical formula of any carbohydrate is CH_2O or $C_xH_{2x}O_x$.

It's All about Carbon, Chemicals, and Reactions

Think of metabolism as the chemistry of life. When students cover this subject in school, they are studying biochemistry.

Biochemistry is built on reactions that occur inside living organisms: plant, animal, and microbe. These reactions differ from the reactions that a chemist runs in a test tube in a laboratory in two ways:

1. Biochemical reactions go forward without needing to be heated up.

2. Biochemical reactions go forward because of the action of specialized proteins called enzymes.

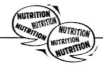

Nutrition Vocabulary

A protein is a string of small nitrogen-containing molecules called amino acids. Certain proteins have the ability to control the chemical reactions of your body. These specialized proteins are called enzymes. Enzymes stop and start the reactions in metabolism and control their speed. Metabolism would not operate at all without enzymes.

Metabolism consists of hundreds of chemical reactions that all follow this basic equation:

$$\text{Substrate A} + \text{Enzyme} \rightarrow \text{Product B} + \text{Enzyme}$$

A substrate is a substance acted upon by an enzyme. After the enzyme tangles with the substrate, it lets go and a new molecule called a product emerges. The enzyme remains unchanged and is ready to repeat the process with a new substrate.

During metabolism, many of these reactions are linked together so that product B becomes a substrate for a different enzyme. Its product in turn becomes the substrate for a third enzyme:

$$\text{Starting Substrate A} + \text{Enzyme 1} \rightarrow \text{B} + \text{Enzyme 2} \rightarrow \text{C} + \text{Enzyme 3} \rightarrow \text{Final Product D}$$

This series of linked reactions is called a metabolic pathway. You are probably already familiar with many important metabolic pathways in nature. These pathways start with a specific chemical and end up with a specific end product (usually a mixture of end products). Here are some of the main metabolic pathways in nature:

➤ Glycolysis: The pathway by which most living things get energy out of the sugar glucose.

➤ Krebs cycle: Also called the tricarboxylic acid cycle, or TCA cycle, this pathway is used by humans and other animals to get energy out of the end products from glycolysis and also from fats and amino acids.

➤ Fermentation: This pathway of certain microbes also follows glycolysis, but it generates energy differently than the Krebs cycle. Fermentation converts sugars into different organic compounds and carbon dioxide without consuming oxygen.

➤ Photosynthesis: This pathway operates in green plants, algae, and microbes containing chlorophyll. It is the route by which carbon dioxide is built into the sugar glucose.

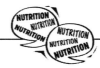

Nutrition Vocabulary

Biochemistry is the study of the chemical reactions that take place in living things. Literally translated, it is the chemistry of life. Since metabolism is a series of many interrelated chemical reactions that take place inside a body, biochemistry and the study of metabolism mean almost the same thing.

Different living things carry out different types of metabolism. Humans are aerobic organisms, meaning our metabolism consists of pathways that consume oxygen while generating energy. This is also true for all other higher forms of animal life. Many microbes have anaerobic metabolism; they cannot use oxygen in their energy-generating pathways.

Since your nutrition is based on oxygen consumption and a diet that provides adequate carbon, we should investigate these pathways in more detail.

Oxygen-consuming organisms are also called respiring organisms. These living things build new body mass and get energy by more than one metabolic pathway that work together as a single mega-pathway known as respiration.

How Respiration Works

Respiration occurs continually in your cells. You know it's working each time you inhale air, which contains 21 percent oxygen (O_2), eat carbon-containing foods, and exhale carbon dioxide (CO_2). With very few exceptions, such as table salt, all foods contain carbon.

Overall, this is what happens inside your cells when they respire:

$$\text{Organic molecules} + O_2 \rightarrow CO_2 + H_2O + \text{Energy} + \text{Heat}$$

Nutrition Morsels

No animal is a perfect nutrition machine that can convert 100 percent of food's energy and nutrients into body mass. Some energy contained in food always gets lost to the cosmos when a meal is digested. This energy loss is in the form of heat. Heat itself is a form of energy. Physicists call it thermal energy. You may notice that you warm up a little after digesting a big meal. This is partly due to the heat energy released when you capture a portion of a food's energy for your own metabolism.

The energy made in respiration is held in a special compound called adenosine triphosphate (ATP). ATP supplies the energy for many of the reactions in metabolism, particularly the anabolic, or body-building, reactions. Like building a house, it takes energy to put up a structure brick by brick.

Three Parts to Respiration

Respiration can be broken down into three main metabolic pathways. Each of these pathways has many side reactions that I will (thankfully) skip over. The three main parts to respiration are:

1. Glycolysis: The pathway that breaks down a six-carbon sugar to two three-carbon products. Glycolysis is sometimes called biology's universal pathway because every organism uses it, from single-celled bacteria to humans. It produces a small number of ATP molecules.

2. Krebs cycle: The products of glycolysis feed into this series of reactions that produces a couple more ATPs and carbon dioxide.

3. Electron transport chain: Another series of enzyme-run reactions in which extra electrons from Krebs cycle reactions get passed through a series of pigments. Most of these pigments are cytochromes. Each cytochrome passes electrons to the next cytochrome in line, and this flow of electrons helps the cell make more ATPs. An oxygen molecule sits at the end of the line and collects the electrons in a final reaction that makes water.

Oxygen is vital to respiration because it collects the electrons that a person's energy-generating pathways produce. If it were not for oxygen, these electrons would build up and stop further reactions. The body therefore needs a steady inflow of oxygen to keep the entire process going forward. The harder you work, the more oxygen you bring into your body to feed those hard-working cells.

The next time you start huffing and puffing on a bicycle or give that treadmill a workout, remember that you're delivering oxygen to the millions of electron transport chains in millions of body cells that are crying out for it.

ATP: Your Energy Currency

You might say that you go to work each day to make money to buy food, and you eat food each day to make another form of currency: ATP. To your body's cells, ATP is far more valuable than a $100 bill. Cells use ATP to run energy-demanding processes. At other times, cells make ATP and hold onto it until it's needed.

The study of how energy flows through a body is called bioenergetics. ATP is a big part of this energy flow. ATP is a simple molecule compared with many other molecules in the body. It consists of three parts:

➤ Adenine: This molecule is also an essential part of your DNA. It is made of carbon, nitrogen, and hydrogen.

➤ Ribose: This sugar, also present in DNA, contains carbon, oxygen, and hydrogen.

➤ Phosphate: This is the simplest part of ATP but the part most important in energy metabolism. It consists of a phosphorus atom attached to four oxygen atoms.

ATP contains three phosphates linked end to end, explaining the *tri* in the name adenosine triphosphate. The bonds that connect the phosphates to each other are the places where the molecule stores its valuable energy. These are called high-energy phosphate bonds.

For reasons that fascinate only biochemists, the bond between the end phosphate and the second phosphate contains the most energy in ATP. When an enzyme transfers this phosphate to another molecule in the body, it also transfers the high-energy phosphate bond. In this way, energy gets passed around from molecule to molecule in cell reactions.

Without studying all the complicated details of bioenergetics, you know at least this: your body cannot generate ATP without a steady supply of carbon, nitrogen, oxygen, hydrogen, and phosphorus. It may not be surprising, then, to learn that along with sulfur, these five elements make up 99 percent of living cells.

How Your Respiration Fits into Earth Biology

Every living thing on Earth is connected through a massive recycling process called the carbon cycle. Since no organism can exist without carbon, each participates in taking in carbon, using it in the body, and then releasing it back into the environment, making it available to other organisms.

You can divide the world of living things into two types: producers and consumers. Photosynthetic organisms play the role of producers. They take in carbon as carbon dioxide and use energy from the Sun to power their anabolism. Consumers, such as cows, humans, and cockroaches, use the organic compounds made by producers to build their own body mass. These organic compounds thus supply consumers with both carbon and energy.

The carbon cycle keeps revolving because photosynthesizers absorb the carbon dioxide exhaled by consumers, and respiring consumers absorb the oxygen released as an end product of photosynthesis. Respiration is therefore an integral piece of the cycle. Earth's carbon moves repeatedly through the reactions that make up respiration and photosynthesis, and around again and again.

Will we ever run out of carbon? It's not likely. Earth contains a massive amount of carbon in fossil fuels, soils and sediments, oceans, and in plant, animal, and microbial cells. Microbes not only store carbon, they also help recycle it by degrading dead plant and animal tissue. Microbes thus help keep the carbon cycle moving every minute. The slowest carbon turnover occurs in what are also Earth's largest carbon deposits: limestone sedimentary rocks.

Nutrition Morsels

Living organisms can be grouped into those that require oxygen for metabolism and those that do not require it. Organisms that live by respiration require oxygen and are called aerobes. Organisms that can get by without both respiration and oxygen are called anaerobes. (Some microbes have a specialized type of respiration called anaerobic respiration, which works without oxygen.)

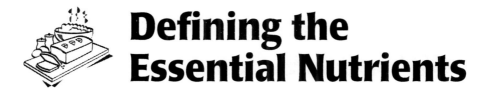

CHAPTER 3

Defining the Essential Nutrients

In This Chapter

➤ The characteristics of an essential nutrient

➤ The difference between macronutrients and micronutrients

➤ Relationship between diet and good nutrition

➤ An introduction to the nutrient groups

In this chapter you will learn about the nutrients you need to maintain your body's metabolism. Foods deliver these nutrients, but no single food contains all the nutrients in the amounts required by the body. To get the right supply and balance of nutrients, you must focus on both the amount of food you eat and the balance of the different types of foods you eat. I'll begin this overview of nutrition by introducing you to the nutrient groups contained in food. In later chapters, you will meet individual nutrients in these groups. Nutritionists call them essential nutrients.

You will also soon see that putting a set value on how much of a nutrient you need can be tricky. If every human body the world over requires the same nutrients, why can't nutritionists agree on the amounts a person needs? In later chapters, you will see how nutrition recommendations are affected by industry and politics, not to mention the harried researcher working away in her lab, waiting for the moment when she can say, "Eureka, I've discovered a new nutrient!"

To understand the state of nutrition today, it's good to remember that several nonscientific factors influence the foods that are marketed to you. Also, nutrition is a science. The goal of science is to uncover new information with each experiment and as new technologies are invented to help scientists in their studies. In other words, what we thought we knew about nutrients fifty years ago is quite different from what we know today. In another fifty years, the story of nutrients will contain many additional layers and nuances.

What Makes an Essential Nutrient Essential?

An essential nutrient is a chemical the body needs but cannot supply in sufficient quantity to support its metabolism. For example, the body needs vitamin D and can actually make its own vitamin D. But often, a person can't make enough vitamin D to maintain good health. In this case, vitamin D is an essential nutrient; the diet must supply the vitamin to make up the difference between the body's needs and what the body can make on its own.

Living things have strict specifications for the types and amounts of carbohydrates, proteins, lipids, vitamins, and minerals that compose their cells. Your cells meet these specifications by taking in essential nutrients contained in food, liberating the carbon, nitrogen, and other elements from the nutrients, and then reassembling these elements into new carbohydrates, proteins, and all other components of the body's cells. Although we constantly build new carbohydrates, proteins, and lipids, most cells tend to use food's vitamins and minerals directly without a lot of reassembly.

Why does the body work hard to break down dietary components only to build carbohydrates, proteins, and other substances all over again? Animals do not directly use the diet's carbohydrates, proteins, and lipids for two reasons:

> ➤ An animal cannot absorb very large molecules, but must first digest them into smaller molecules in order to get them through the intestinal lining and into the bloodstream.

> ➤ The body evolved in a way that has very specific requirements for the exact structure of its carbohydrates, proteins, and lipids. Since the digestive tract breaks down these three nutrients anyway, the body's cells might as well put the elements back together again in an arrangement that best serves the body.

Nutrition Morsels

The USDA is responsible for overseeing the United States' agricultural products and agriculture business. Because of this role, the USDA also oversees the nation's nutrition policies. These policies relate to the types of foods Americans eat or should be eating, and the safety of those foods. The USDA is involved in nutrition education programs, the nutrient requirements based on scientific studies, guidelines on the food groups supplying these nutrients, and food inspections for potential contamination or other hazards.

Three organizations within the USDA handle most of these responsibilities: the Center for Nutrition Policy and Promotion (CNPP), the Food and Nutrition Service (FNS), and the Food Safety and Inspection Service (FSIS).

Macronutrients and Micronutrients

A well-balanced human diet typically supplies plenty of carbohydrates, proteins, and lipids. That's a good thing because the body needs a lot of these nutrients to run metabolism.

The nutrients that are used by the body in large amounts are called macronutrients. The body needs these nutrients in the highest amounts, and, not coincidentally, a human diet supplies them in the largest quantities. The human diet, after all, evolved as humans evolved to provide us with the nutrients we need and in the correct proportions.

The macronutrients are:

> ➤ Carbohydrates: These are compounds made of carbon, hydrogen, and oxygen. These nutrients are the main carbon and energy sources for your body.

> ➤ Proteins: These are nitrogen-containing nutrients that supply amino acids so that your cells can reassemble them into new proteins that the body uses. Proteins make up body tissues, control the immune system, make you move, and regulate the body's metabolism and reproduction.

> ➤ Fats and other lipids: These substances are mainly carbon and hydrogen and are essential in energy storage and as components of cells and cell membranes.

> ➤ Calcium: Critical in nerve and muscle function and in development of bone.

> ➤ Phosphorus: Critical in energy metabolism.

➤ Sulfur: Part of proteins, sulfur is essential in many enzymes and structural proteins.

➤ Sodium: Critical in nerve signal transmission and other types of cell communication.

➤ Potassium: Plays a role complementary to sodium's in cell communication.

➤ Chlorine: A component of stomach acid, a participant in nerve function, and an electrolyte that helps balance blood chemistry.

➤ Magnesium: An essential component for many enzymes. Helps in bone formation, and acts in nerve function.

All of the above macronutrients, except sulfur and magnesium, should be in the daily diet in gram amounts. Usually, dietary protein automatically gives you enough sulfur, so you never have to worry about getting enough sulfur by itself. An adult's magnesium requirement is about 0.5 gram a day. This is less than the other macronutrients, but much more than the requirement for micronutrients.

Nutritionists have recently begun to include two additional macronutrients for good nutrition: fiber and water. I'll discuss fiber and water in more detail in separate chapters but will also introduce them to you here.

Nutrition Vocabulary

An electrolyte is an element able to separate into positively and negatively charged components. These charged forms of the element then help conduct electrical currents in the body. The main electrolytes are sodium (Na) as Na^+, potassium (K) as K^+, and chlorine (Cl) as chloride, Cl^-.

Micronutrients are nutrients used by the body in tiny amounts. They are:

➤ All vitamins.

➤ Micro-minerals needed for good health, but in very low concentrations in the diet. Iron and zinc are examples of micro-minerals.

You need micronutrients in miniscule amounts, such as micrograms (μg) per day or much less. A microgram is 0.000001 gram (g).

Because micronutrient requirements are very small, you can usually meet them by ingesting a good balance of the carbohydrate, fat, and protein foods. The micronutrients come along for the ride!

Nutrition Morsels

A gram is a measure of weight like a pound is a measure of weight. A chemist will tell you that a gram equals the weight of one cubic centimeter (cc) of water. Picture the size of a sugar cube. A cube of water about this size would equal 1 gram. Another way to think of a gram is to picture about 1/6 teaspoon of salt.

The Evolution of the Western Diet

Nutrition has become a complicated subject. Primitive humans went on the hunt when they were hungry. They slaughtered an ox or a rabbit, pulled fish from oceans and streams, and collected roots and fruit to complete their meal. The energy expended to hunt and gather food had to add up to less than the energy contained in their food, or else they would become emaciated and might even starve. So ancient nutrient requirements were simple: eat enough to maintain the energy levels needed for the next day's hunting and gathering.

Nutrition has not changed at all since humans evolved on Earth. We must still eat enough food to give us sufficient energy to hunt (for parking spaces, good schools, new clients, and golden investment opportunities) and gather (grocery shop, cash a paycheck, buy a new house, and pick up the kids at soccer).

Diets, however, have changed dramatically over the centuries. Early societies depended on the foods available to their communities or through occasional trading with nearby settlements. But industrialization changed the way people ate and where they got their foods. As global commerce expanded to its modern state, diets changed too.

Nutrition Vocabulary

The noun *diet* refers to the main types of foods and drinks that a person normally eats. The verb *diet* does not, however, mean "to eat." In Western culture, to diet is to reduce your food intake with the goal of losing weight. A person might further confuse these terms by saying, "I'm on a diet," to explain that they are trying to eat less and lose weight.

In this book, diet is the main foods that a person consumes. Dieting is the act of reducing food intake for the purpose of losing weight.

The nutrient requirements of the human body remain the same as they have always been, even before anyone had invented a science called nutrition. In industrialized places, however, the foods eaten to meet these requirements differ markedly from the fresh fruit and vegetables and newly slaughtered game animals that made up early civilization's diet.

I will use the term *Western diet* to describe the types of foods that are popular in most industrialized places in the world. I'll further narrow this description to North America to help eliminate cultural influences on diet in various parts of the world. This Western diet has the following characteristics:

➤ The variety and amount of foods are excellent, but people often do not choose the foods correctly to produce a balanced diet.

➤ Energy intake, measured in calories, is often too much for a person's energy needs.

➤ Fiber content is too low, and fat and carbohydrate content is too high.

➤ Too much emphasis has been placed on vitamin and mineral supplements and not enough on a balanced diet that can provide these nutrients.

➤ The salt, sugar, and/or alcohol content tends to be too high.

➤ Many dietary choices are made for reasons related to emotion, stress, habit, marketing, or social influences, and less related to good nutrition.

The Western diet also has three hallmarks that developed since the Industrial Revolution in the nineteenth century. The first hallmark relates to a high proportion of processed foods in the diet. The second relates to how foods are produced and distributed. Today, most foods are produced in a small number of facilities in the United States, and then distributed by truck to vast points all over the map.

The third hallmark combines the other two: Western diets include a high proportion of meals prepared outside the home. This ranges from fast food joints to restaurants that tout only the freshest local ingredients.

Regardless of the characteristics of your particular diet, you can achieve good nutrition. It begins first by understanding nutrient requirements and second by understanding the essential nutrients.

The Meaning of Nutrient Requirements

The terminology used by nutritionists to guide you in meeting your nutrient needs varies depending on what country you live in. The United States and Canada use the term *recommended daily allowance* (RDA) to describe a nutrient's requirements for a person of a certain age and body weight. Europe and the World Health Organization (WHO) have adopted slightly different terms. The European Communities (EC) use the term *population reference intake* (PRI) and WHO uses *recommended nutrient intake* (RNI).

Nutrition Vocabulary

A recommended daily allowance (RDA) is a daily average of the amount of a nutrient needed to protect an individual against deficiency. In other words, an RDA tells you the amount of a nutrient that one person should consume daily.

Since the RDA is an average based on a larger population of people, any individual might require a certain nutrient at levels a little above the RDA or a little below the RDA. Most people's diets fluctuate from day to day, so falling below the RDA on any particular day will not doom you. All nutrient recommendations are based on ranges of nutrient intake to cover as wide a range of different shapes, sizes, and ages of people as possible.

Other types of nutrient guidelines you might see in nutrition resources are:

➤ Dietary reference value (DRV), dietary reference intake (DRI), nutrient intake value (NIV), and population reference intake (PRI): All of these are equivalent to the RDA and might be used in different parts of the world.

➤ Estimated average requirement (EAR): Amount of a nutrient that meets the nutritional needs of half of any particular group of people, such as females, children under six years old, or people older than seventy.

➤ Adequate intake (AI): A daily level of intake for a nutrient for which insufficient research data exists to assign this nutrient an RDA.

➤ Tolerable upper intake level (UL): The highest amount of a nutrient you can consume daily without causing harm to your health.

➤ Estimated energy requirement (EER): An energy level needed to maintain the energy use of an average person in a specific stage of life.

Proteins, Carbohydrates, and Fats—Telling Them Apart

Proteins, carbohydrates, and fats make up the bulk of your diet, and you need them in the largest amounts. You body is mainly protein, carbohydrate, fat, and water.

Proteins are strings of amino acids linked end to end and then folded up in a specific pattern. They contain carbon, hydrogen, oxygen, nitrogen, and usually sulfur. Proteins serve your cells as a ready source of nitrogen, which is needed for making new proteins as well as DNA and other components of your genetics.

Carbohydrates contain a specific ratio of carbon, hydrogen, and oxygen. This nutrient group contains the sugars, starches, and fibers. Starches are long strands of sugars linked together and contain many branches. Sugars and starches are the body's main energy sources. Sugars also appear on the outside of cells, often connected to a protein, and serve in cell-to-cell communication. (A protein that has a sugar attached to it is called a glycoprotein. The prefix *glyco* stands for sugar.)

A fat is a compound made mainly of carbon and hydrogen with only a small amount of oxygen. Fats serve as your body's long-term energy storage. Fat also makes up adipose tissue, which helps protect internal organs and insulates the body. Fats belong to a larger class of substances called lipids.

Lipids are substances that do not dissolve in water and play varied roles in the body. In addition to being involved in energy storage, lipids provide the framework for vitamin D and some hormones, and are important in cell membranes. In addition to fats, lipids include oils and sterols. The main sterol in animal bodies is cholesterol. (Plants do not contain cholesterol.)

Meet the Vitamins

A vitamin is a chemical needed in the diet in very small amounts (micronutrient) and helps regulate specific steps in metabolism. Vitamins participate in these steps by aiding the action of enzymes. When vitamins team up with enzymes, the vitamin is said to play the part of a coenzyme.

Vitamins are divided into two groups: water-soluble and fat-soluble. The water-soluble vitamins are the B vitamins and vitamin C. In general, the B vitamins are integral in energy-generating steps in the body and in blood chemistry. The B vitamins are:

➤ Thiamin (B_1)

➤ Riboflavin (B_2)

➤ Niacin

➤ Pyridoxine (B_6)

➤ Folic acid

➤ Cobalamin (B_{12})

➤ Pantothenic acid

➤ Biotin

Vitamin C has various diverse jobs in the body, many of which involve protecting tissue from chemical harm.

The fat-soluble vitamins are vitamins A, D, E, and K. Each of these vitamins has specific and different roles in the body.

As a general rule, B vitamins must be replaced quicker than fat-soluble vitamins because the kidneys excrete B vitamins in urine. The body can store fat-soluble vitamins in adipose tissue. For this reason, you are more likely to accumulate high levels of fat-soluble vitamins in your body if you take vitamin supplements than water-soluble vitamins, which the body readily excretes.

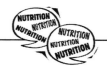

Nutrition Vocabulary

A coenzyme is a chemical that combines with an inactive enzyme to activate the enzyme so it can carry out its function in a cell.

Meet the Minerals

A mineral is any chemical element that helps the body's chemical reactions go forward, and it may also play a role in forming the body's structures. Unlike carbohydrates, proteins, fats, and vitamins, minerals are not organic; they do not contain carbon. Minerals are called inorganic chemicals.

Nutritionists divide minerals into two groups:

➤ Macro-minerals: The macronutrients calcium, phosphorus, sulfur, sodium, potassium, chlorine, and magnesium.

➤ Micro-minerals or trace elements: All other minerals required by the body in very low amounts. The micro-minerals known so far are chromium, cobalt, copper, fluorine, iodine, iron, manganese, molybdenum, selenium, and zinc.

Micro-minerals have varied roles in the body. One essential role is as a cofactor for enzymes.

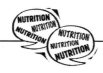

Nutrition Vocabulary

A cofactor is a mineral or other non-vitamin that binds to a specific region of a protein to enable that protein to work. If the protein happens to be an enzyme, the binding of enzyme and cofactor activates the enzyme, similar to how vitamin coenzymes activate enzymes.

The Other Nutrients

Water and fiber have been categorized as nutrients too because of their importance to good health. In the case of water, no chemical reaction in the body can take place without it, so water can perhaps be considered the most essential of essential nutrients.

Fiber is important in proper functioning of the digestive tract and may affect nutrient absorption. The roles of water and fiber in good nutrition will be mentioned repeatedly in this book.

CHAPTER 4

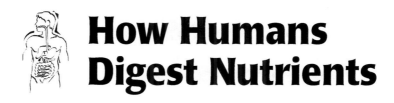

How Humans Digest Nutrients

In This Chapter

➤ The human digestive tract and their functions

➤ The main digestive enzymes

➤ Phases of food processing by the body

➤ Non-digestive-tract organs that help with digestion

In this chapter you journey through the digestive tract. Picture yourself as a morsel of food that enters the mouth, gets chewed up and swallowed, and then takes a ride through a cauldron of acids, a tunnel overrun with millions of bacteria, and then a slow chug toward the exit door. So much of nutrition takes place before any nutrient ever gets absorbed into the body that this subject deserves its own chapter.

Here, you will meet the main organs that break down your food so its products can be absorbed into your bloodstream. You will also learn how certain organs of the body support digestion.

Almost every organ of the digestive tract plays a unique and crucial part in digestion. You might be able to survive if any one of these organs were removed or lost its ability to function, but it wouldn't be easy. Good nutrition rests on a healthy digestive tract from beginning to end.

Your Digestive Tract

Your digestive tract is a tube that runs from the mouth to the anus. Although you might think of food as being inside your body after you swallow it, the digestive tract is outside your body. Only substances that get absorbed through the skin or the mucosa are truly inside your body.

The digestive tract contains two main components that impact nutrition: bacteria and digestive enzymes. Bacteria are single-celled organisms that feast on the foods you ingest. They release a variety of enzymes that digest your meal. The bacteria absorb the end products of digestion for their own use. But during this process, they also help you by breaking down tough-to-digest materials such as dietary fibers.

Your body also releases digestive enzymes. Many are identical to the ones produced by the bacteria. These enzymes help digest foods, and they also break down dead bacterial cells. So the bacteria not only help in nutrition when they're alive, they also help when they are dead. The body gets a significant amount of its nutrients from dead bacterial cells that have been digested by body enzymes secreted into the digestive tract.

Digestive Enzymes

Digestive enzymes perform the lion's share of food breakdown. Specific enzymes target specific components of food so that several enzymes attack a meal at the same time. The list below illustrates that some enzymes are released from different points along the digestive tract. The enzymes that first begin the breakdown of ingested food are:

> ➤ Salivary amylase: In the mouth's saliva, this enzyme degrades polysaccharides, such as starch, into smaller strands of sugars.

> ➤ Pancreatic amylase: Secreted by the pancreas, this enzyme enters the small intestines and continues the breakdown of partially digested polysaccharides.

> ➤ Trypsin and chymotrypsin: Both enzymes come from the pancreas and degrade polypeptides into shorter strands of amino acids, called peptides.

> ➤ Nucleases: These also come from the pancreas and break down nucleic acids.

> ➤ Lipases: Yet another group of enzymes from the pancreas, these degrade fats and need the help of bile salts to work at their best.

> ➤ Pepsin: The stomach secretes this enzyme, which degrades proteins into polypeptides.

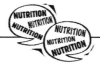

Nutrition Vocabulary

Bile is a mixture of substances made in the liver, stored in the gallbladder, and secreted into the intestines to help with fat digestion. Bile contains bile salts, which allow bile to act as a detergent inside the intestines. This detergent activity makes fats easier to attack by lipase enzymes. By working together, bile salts and lipases enhance your ability to digest fats from food.

Why are fats more difficult to digest than other nutrients? Because they are not soluble in water and your intestines are an aqueous environment, that is, one that is filled mainly with water. Bile is also essential in the absorption of vitamins D and E.

After the main digestive enzymes, listed above, attack the big components of food—starch, protein, nucleic acid, and fat—another set of enzymes steps up to further break down the materials into units the body can absorb:

➤ Disaccharidases: These enzymes cleave disaccharides (molecules made of two sugars) into single sugars.

➤ Carboxypeptidase and dipeptidase: These enzymes break down peptides into individual amino acids.

➤ Nucleotidases, nucleosidases, and phosphatases: These three types of enzymes work together to degrade nucleic acids into their component sugars, nitrogen-containing bases, and phosphate structures.

Most of the above enzymes are secreted by the small intestines. The exception is carboxypeptidase, which is made by the pancreas.

The Phases of Food Processing

Overall, your digestive tract is responsible for four phases of food processing. One or more organs of the digestive tract carry out these phases:

1. Ingestion: The act of eating is the first stage of food processing and is carried out in higher animals by the mouth.

2. Digestion: This is the second phase of food processing and comprises the breaking down of food into smaller molecules that the body can absorb. Enzymes secreted by the body and by your intestinal bacteria digest food. This phase occurs mainly in the mouth and the small intestines. The stomach also helps out to a lesser extent by secreting strong acids.

3. Absorption: The small molecules produced in food digestion get absorbed by the cells lining the intestines.

4. Elimination: In this final phase, all undigested material is excreted from the body via the large intestine (colon or large bowel) and exits through the anus.

The Mouth and Upper Digestive Tract

The mouth carries out two important steps in food processing. It is the place where food gets masticated, where the action of teeth and jaw muscles physically cuts, smashes, and grinds your food. During all this destruction, the mouth squirts saliva onto the food to make it easier to swallow. Saliva delivers the second step in food processing: it adds amylase enzymes to begin the breakdown of carbohydrates.

A masticated piece of food gets shaped in the mouth by the action of the roof of the mouth and the tongue to form a bolus. This is simply a ball of food that moves farther along the digestive tract when you swallow.

The upper digestive tract has three main parts, the pharynx (throat), epiglottis, and esophagus. The epiglottis is a flap that closes the opening to your windpipe (the glottis) every time you swallow. This action prevents food from entering your respiratory tract, which could lead to choking. (When a small piece of food accidentally enters the glottis, you experience the uncomfortable situation known as . . . "It went down the wrong pipe!")

The esophagus carries each bolus of food from the throat to the stomach. It does this by creating waves of muscle contractions that are collectively called peristalsis. Peristalsis pushes food through the digestive tract.

Nutrition Morsels

Choking occurs when your swallowing reflex does not close the windpipe in time to allow food to pass by. Instead, some food or liquid enters the windpipe and blocks airflow to your lungs. The body quickly responds by activating a second reflex: coughing. Vigorous coughing can usually push out the obstruction, but if it doesn't, choking can be fatal.

The Stomach

Food passes from the esophagus to the stomach through an opening called the cardiac orifice. Once inside the stomach, food undergoes some digestion due to the action of very strong gastric juices. This liquid is mainly hydrochloric acid and has about the same acidity as battery acid! How does the acid keep from eating right through the stomach lining? The stomach's main protection comes from mucus, which is secreted by the cells lining the organ and protects the stomach from digesting itself.

Gastric juice is instrumental in the first step of protein digestion. During the time proteins remain in the stomach, the acids do two things. First, they denature the proteins, meaning the acid causes the proteins to relax and unfold. Then, the acid activates the enzyme pepsin, which begins to cleave the unfolded protein.

The stomach lining contains two types of cells. Chief cells secrete the inactivated form of pepsin. By storing this enzyme in an inactive form, the enzyme cannot digest the proteins in the very cell that makes it. Parietal cells are dispersed among the chief cells. These cells secrete the hydrochloric acid that activates the pepsin.

The stomach wall contains many deep folds, and the entire organ can stretch to accommodate about 2 quarts of food and liquid but normally holds about 1 quart. This comes in handy when sitting down to a Thanksgiving meal but also works against us when we are trying to lose weight by eating less. About every 20 seconds, the stomach contracts to mix whatever food is inside it. This helps with digestion but in an empty stomach the contraction causes a slight pain known as hunger pangs.

Physiologists give the name *acid chyme* to the food that has been thoroughly mixed with stomach enzymes and acid. Acid chyme is the material that moves on to the small intestines.

The Intestines

The intestines consist of the small intestine and the large intestine. Acid chyme goes from the stomach to the first part of the small intestine through an opening called the pyloric sphincter. A sphincter is a circular opening controlled by a muscle that opens and closes it.

The small intestine is the main site of digestion and nutrient absorption. Most of your digested carbohydrates, proteins, fats, vitamins, and minerals get absorbed here. The small intestine consists of three sections:

1. Duodenum: The first 10 inches or so of the small intestine where acid chyme mixes with digestive enzymes, and a major part of food digestion occurs

2. Jejunum: A stretch of intestine about 8 feet long that is constantly contracting. This section is a site of continued digestion and a significant amount of nutrient absorption

3. Ileum: The last part of the small intestine that continues the absorption process

The human small intestine holds about 4 quarts of watery material.

The ileum connects to the large intestine by another sphincter. The large intestine's role is mainly to recover water by absorbing it through the colon wall. Together, the small and large intestines can reabsorb about 90 percent of the water that first enters the duodenum.

The large intestine also harbors an enormous population of bacteria that play a role in nutrition by making B vitamins and amino acids. Some of these can be absorbed through the intestinal wall. These microbes also help break down certain hard-to-digest carbohydrates from foods.

The rectum, where feces is formed, is the last part of the digestive tract. The anus is a sphincter that separates the rectum from the outside world.

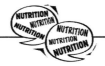

Nutrition Vocabulary

Peristalsis is any action in nature characterized by waves of muscle contractions. In the digestive tract, these muscles are part of your involuntary muscle system, or muscles that work on their own without you thinking about them. Peristalsis serves to move partially digested food from the esophagus to the end of the digestive tract, the rectum.

Organs that Support Digestion

Several organs and hormones support digestion. Although these organs are not part of the digestive tract, proper digestion cannot occur without them. These organs are the liver, gallbladder, and pancreas. The nervous system and musculature also play a supportive role by controlling the sphincters and contractile muscles of the digestive tract.

The Liver

The liver acts mainly to process many of the products of digestion. A significant portion of the blood that receives absorbed nutrients from the digestive tract goes straight to the liver.

Liver cells (hepatocytes) remove excess nutrients, especially glucose, from the blood before the blood circulates to the rest of the body. The liver assembles individual glucose sugars into a large storage form called glycogen. The liver's glycogen thus serves as an important energy storage point for carbon and energy because glucose is the body's main carbon and energy source.

The liver also breaks down any excess amino acids absorbed by the intestines. The body uses many amino acids right away for making new proteins. But some amino acids are left over. The liver removes the nitrogen from these excess amino acids and turns it into the waste product ammonia (NH_3). The liver cells then put two ammonias together to make urea, which it then dumps into the bloodstream. The blood carries urea to the kidneys for elimination. The rest of the amino acid molecule can be fed into either of two metabolic pathways:

1. Glycolysis and Krebs cycle for generating energy

2. Gluconeogenesis for building glucose to be stored in glycogen

The liver keeps everything in balance. Liver cells convert carbohydrates to fats, amino acids to carbohydrates and fats, and fats into carbohydrates and other cell constituents. Meanwhile, the liver clears toxins from blood and degrades alcohol, which is also toxic at high levels. Toxins could be any harmful substance produced by an infection or your normal metabolism, a drug, a chemical from the environment, or an excess of a certain nutrient.

Last but not least, the liver decomposes used red blood cells and removes the pigment from them. This pigment, called bilirubin, gets eliminated from the body with the feces. If the liver is damaged, the pigments build up in the blood and skin. This condition is known as jaundice.

The Gallbladder

The gallbladder is a small sac situated next to the liver. Bile ducts drain bile from the liver and carry it to the gallbladder, which concentrates and stores the bile. The presence of fats in a meal induces the gallbladder to contract. The contraction then pushes the bile through a duct leading to the duodenum.

The composition of bile secreted from the gallbladder is about 92 percent water, 6 percent bile salts, 0.3 percent bilirubin, 0.3 percent lecithin, and 0.3 percent or more each of cholesterol and fats. Bile also contains high amounts of ions of sodium, potassium, calcium, chlorine, and bicarbonate, which help emulsify fats during fat digestion. Here's how some of these bile components help in fat emulsification and digestion:

➤ Bile salts: These substances are all derived from cholesterol. In the intestines, they coat fat droplets, which helps keep the fat suspended in the watery conditions. This mixing of fat and water is part of fat emulsification.

➤ Lecithin: This detergent-like substance affects the boundary between a fat and water, which makes it easier for lipases to digest the fat.

Fats cannot be absorbed through the intestinal lining until they have been sufficiently dispersed into tiny droplets called micelles. Only the action of bile salts, lecithin, and the ions in bile make micelle formation possible.

The Pancreas

Your pancreas helps your overall health in two ways: by secreting digestive enzymes into the duodenum and by producing hormones that regulate blood glucose levels.

Pancreatic enzymes help in the digestion of carbohydrates, proteins, lipids, and nucleic acids. About 90 percent of pancreatic cells are involved in enzyme secretion. Three types of hormone-producing cells are dispersed throughout pancreatic tissue. They congregate in clusters called pancreatic islets, or the islets of Langerhans. These cells produce three different hormones:

1. Insulin: Functions to lower blood glucose levels from an optimum concentration. This hormone is produced by islet beta cells.

2. Glucagon: Functions to raise blood glucose levels; produced by alpha cells.

3. Somatostatin: Functions to control the levels of the other two hormones.

Nutrition Morsels

Several hormones help regulate how your body responds to food after you have taken your first bite of a meal. The hormone gastrin is produced by the stomach and stimulates the production of gastric juices when you begin eating. When amino acids or certain fats enter the duodenum, this organ releases cholecystokinin, which stimulates the pancreas to release its own battery of digestive enzymes.

The duodenum also makes the hormone secretin, which stimulates the pancreas to release sodium bicarbonate. This material helps neutralize the acids in acid chyme.

Finally, the duodenum secretes enterogastrone, which slows peristalsis and stops the stomach's acid secretion. Foods high in fats are the trigger for enterogastrone release.

Eliminating Wastes

Getting rid of waste is as important to good nutrition as consuming a balanced diet. The digestive tract cannot process more food and get adequate nutrients and energy from your diet if you cannot eliminate the undigested portion of your diet. Similarly, the end products of metabolism must be excreted from the body so that they do not build up to toxic levels. Thus, the colon, specifically the rectum and anus, eliminates undigested food, and the kidneys eliminate metabolized substances.

The Colon

This portion of the large intestine stores feces until the body eliminates this waste. One or more times a day, the large intestine undergoes strong contractions that a person perceives as an urge to defecate.

The Kidneys

The kidneys contain an intricate network of vessels and tubes that filter wastes out of blood to produce urine. Each of your body's kidneys contains more than a million tiny blood-cleaning units called nephrons. Urine is produced in the nephron, which drains into a vessel leading to the ureter that in turn enables urine to flow to the bladder.

In addition to processing the wastes in blood for excretion, the kidneys also maintain the body's blood volume, correct the blood's balance of water and salts, and adjust the amount of acidity in blood.

PART TWO

Powering Your Body

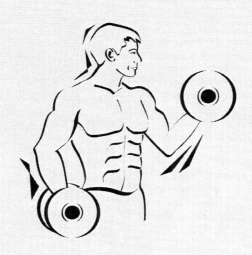

CHAPTER 5

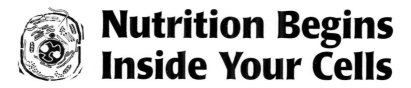

Nutrition Begins Inside Your Cells

> ## In This Chapter
>
> ➤ The role of cells in nutrition
>
> ➤ How nutrients get into your cells
>
> ➤ Oxygen, respiration, energy, and electrons

In this chapter you follow a nutrient into the most basic unit that makes up your body: the cell. Eating and breathing are the ways you bring life-giving substances into to your body. Do you ever think about where the food, water, and oxygen go after you have taken them inside?

Nutrition is part of a bigger subject in biology called human physiology. You are an organism; so is every other human, every other animal, tiny microbe, and all plants and fungi.

Excluding the simple microbes, every organism is a collection of organ systems that work together to keep the body alive. Organ systems are made of individual organs. For example, the digestive system consists of the mouth, esophagus, stomach, intestines, and so on. Each organ consists of different types of tissues that have discrete jobs. Tissue is a collection of the same type of cells. To understand nutrition, you really need to know what happens inside cells.

What Cells Do

A cell is the basic unit upon which all living things are built. An amoeba consists of only one cell. The human body, by contrast, contains about 10 trillion cells. The job of good nutrition is to supply each cell with the amount and variety of chemicals it needs to carry out its metabolism. When you order a cheeseburger and fries, select a morsel of sushi, or punch the button on a vending machine for a bag of chips, you are ultimately preparing to feed your cells.

Cells take in chemicals (nutrients) and employ enzymes to build new cell constituents out of these chemicals. By making new cells, a person grows, strengthens the skeleton, enlarges muscle, fights infection, repairs injury, and reproduces.

Inside almost every cell of the body, the following activities are occurring at a faster or slower pace, depending on your specific needs at the moment:

> ➤ Building protein from amino acids or breaking down protein to release amino acids

> ➤ Storing energy as glucose in glycogen or breaking down glycogen to get energy

> ➤ Making a long-term energy storage form as fat in adipose tissue or breaking down those fats for energy

> ➤ Replicating DNA as cells divide to make new cells

> ➤ Building cell constituents, called organelles, out of proteins, carbohydrates, and fats, or deconstructing them to liberate the proteins, carbohydrates, and fats for energy

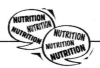

Nutrition Vocabulary

Organelles are structures inside cells that have particular functions. Cells can have about fifteen different types of organelles; most contain about ten. Among their many functions, organelles maintain your genetic material, run energy-generating steps of metabolism, produce cellular products, transport materials into and out of the cell, and destroy certain unwanted materials such as an infectious virus. Many specific steps in nutrient use take place in specific organelles.

In addition to all of these activities, specialized cells have additional jobs to perform. For example, endocrine cells make and secrete hormones, nerve cells transmit signals through the body, and muscle cells make your body move.

Cells cannot function without a reliable supply of the nutrients they need.

Cell Membranes

Nutrients enter cells when they cross the outer barrier of the cell, called its membrane. Membranes are one of the several different types of cell organelles.

A membrane is a pliable fluidlike assembly of proteins and lipids. Lipids make up the main structure of the membrane. The lipids are oriented in membranes so that their water-attracting portions are on the membrane's outer and inner surfaces. In between these two surfaces lies the water-repelling portion of the lipids. The entire assembly looks a little like a peanut butter sandwich.

Various proteins lie interspersed in the membrane lipids. Some of the proteins extend all the way across the membrane and touch both the cell exterior and its interior; other proteins go only halfway across the membrane.

Membranes also contain an occasional cholesterol in between the lipids. Cholesterol keeps membranes from being too squishy and from hardening at low temperatures.

The outer surface of all biological membranes holds an array of complex substances called glycolipids and glycoproteins. Since the prefix *glyco* refers to any sugar, you can see that glycolipids are lipids with a sugar molecule attached to them, and glycoproteins are proteins with a sugar molecule attached. These substances play an essential role in allowing cells in the body to recognize each other, especially so that cells of the same type can team up to form tissue.

Membrane Transport of Nutrients

Different nutrients get across a cell's membrane by different mechanisms. The main factor in how a cell determines which mechanism to use relates to energy. Cells try to minimize the energy they must spend to get a nutrient inside.

Various nutrients cross a cell's membrane by these main transport mechanisms:

➤ Diffusion: The drifting of small molecules across the membrane without the need for expending any energy. Water and ions use diffusion to get into cells.

➤ Facilitated diffusion: A type of low-energy transport similar to diffusion with the addition of a membrane protein to help the nutrient get across. The cell uses this method for taking in some amino acids.

➤ Active transport: In this transport mechanism, the cell must expend energy to carry sugars, amino acids, fats, and the building blocks of nucleic acids across the membrane. This mechanism is also aided by proteins that are part of the cell's membrane.

➤ Bulk transport: In this mechanism, the cell takes in very large nutrients called macromolecules by enveloping an entire nutrient with its membrane. Some large vitamins, such as vitamin B_{12}, may require this type of transport.

Nutrition Vocabulary

Many nutrients are large chemicals called macromolecules, which must be broken down into smaller molecules before the intestines can absorb them and put them into the bloodstream.

Macromolecules are often made of two or more smaller molecules linked together by a chemical bond. Polysaccharides, proteins, nucleic acids, cholesterol, and some vitamins are examples of macromolecules found in foods. Vitamins are distinct among macromolecules because the intestines absorb them whole rather than break them into pieces.

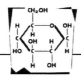

The Chemistry of Nutrition

Do you think you have an electric personality? If so, there's a chemical reason. Energy-yielding reactions in the body operate because of the transfer of electrons from one chemical to the next.

An electron is a tiny negatively charged component of an atom. An atom is the smallest basic unit in chemistry, just as cells are the basic unit of all biological organisms. Atoms are composed of protons, neutrons, and electrons. The positive charge of protons usually cancels the negative charge of the atom's electrons. Neutrons are neutral; they carry no charge.

Electrons orbit the atom's nucleus, which is packed with all the atom's protons and neutrons. An atom therefore looks a bit like our solar system of planets orbiting the Sun. In your body, electrons are a key component of energy metabolism. As chemicals hand electrons to each other in the electron transport chain, some energy is released. This energy goes into making new ATP.

Oxygen

We do not think of oxygen as a nutrient because we get it from breathing using our respiratory system rather than from food. Yet oxygen is like a nutrient in that the body cannot produce it, so we must have a steady supply of it from an outside source.

Nutrition is inextricably linked to how the body uses oxygen. Oxygen is a component of every nutrient except the minerals. Oxygen also plays a pivotal role in chemical reactions of the body called redox reactions—*redox* is short for reduction and oxidation. Many of the steps in anabolism and catabolism are redox reactions.

Reduction reactions are those in which electrons are added to a molecule. In the opposite reaction, oxidation, electrons are taken away from a molecule. Often in biology, an oxidation reaction also involves the addition of oxygen. For example, in the following equation, the gas methane (CH_4) is being oxidized to produce carbon dioxide (CO_2):

$$CH_4 + O_2 \rightarrow CO_2 + H_2O + Energy$$

Oxygen gas also serves us by being an integral part of the energy-generating processes known as respiration.

Respiration

Respiration is nature's most efficient energy-generating type of catabolism. A simple way to view respiration is as a pathway for converting the energy held in organic compounds to energy the body can use:

Organic compounds + Oxygen ➔ Carbon dioxide + Water + Energy

A chemist might rewrite the above equation like this:

$$C_6H_{12}O_6 + 6\,O_2 \rightarrow 6\,CO_2 + 6\,H_2O + ATP + Heat$$

The body uses the ATPs for various maintenance activities and work. The heat that is released by respiration warms the body a bit but much of it is lost to the environment.

Nutrition Morsels

In biology, work is any action that requires energy input. Cells perform three different types of work: mechanical, transport, and chemical. Mechanical work is movement, such as the contraction of a muscle. Transport work is the process of moving substances into or out of cells, such as the absorption of glucose. Chemical work relates to any reactions inside cells that require energy to proceed. For example, building new proteins is an energy-demanding process, so the cell views this as work.

To produce all the ATPs they need to do work, cells run three processes. These processes are glycolysis, the Krebs cycle, and the electron transport chain. Each consists of a series of chemical reactions, most of which are redox reactions. Each reaction uses carbon chemicals, so each process relies on a steady input of dietary carbon. This carbon comes mainly from the carbohydrates you eat.

Individual reactions in respiration are run by enzymes. Therefore, the proteins in your diet are essential in supplying the amino acids your cells need to make these specific enzymes.

Many of the enzymes that control glycolysis, the Krebs cycle, and electron transport require helper substances called coenzymes and cofactors. Vitamins are the body's coenzymes;

several minerals play the role of cofactors. This is why your daily intake of vitamins and minerals is so important in order for you to feel energized.

Where do all those electrons get transported to during respiration? Oxygen molecules line up at the end of the electron transport chain and grab them. The oxygen then goes into a new molecule of water, becoming the *O* in H_2O. The body uses this water in various ways and excretes any excess through the kidneys.

Adenosine Triphosphate (ATP)

The goal of glycolysis, the Krebs cycle, and electron transport is to make ATP. This is the substance that carries energy in your cells and that your cells use like money whenever they need to pay an energy debt.

It takes energy for a muscle cell (called a muscle fiber) to contract. The cell pays the energy cost with ATP. Similarly, the cell pays a toll each time it brings glucose, amino acids, and other nutrients across its membrane. It pays this toll with ATP. Think of all the nutrients you must ingest to give your cells the ingredients to make new ATPs:

➤ Carbon: Mainly from carbohydrates but also supplied in proteins and fats

➤ Nitrogen: From proteins

➤ Oxygen: Mainly from carbohydrates

➤ Hydrogen: From carbohydrates, proteins, and fats

➤ Phosphorus: Comes with foods that are also good protein sources, such as dairy products and eggs, meat and fish, nuts and some seeds.

CHAPTER 6

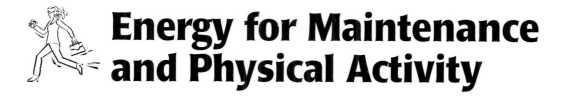 Energy for Maintenance and Physical Activity

> ### In This Chapter
>
> ➤ Ways to measure food energy
> ➤ Components of the body's energy balance
> ➤ Factors that affect appetite, hunger, and food intake
> ➤ Everyone's food energy requirements

In this chapter energy is the main topic of discussion. All nutrition is aimed at giving your body the energy it needs to move, digest more food, think, grow, reproduce, and simply maintain.

Over a certain period of time, you must ingest enough food to supply energy for two needs. First, you need enough energy to maintain your body, a little bit like keeping a car idling. This maintenance is called basal metabolism. Once you have given your body enough energy to keep the engine idling, you'll probably want extra energy to supply the second need, which is physical activity.

This chapter describes your body's energy needs, the ways your body controls the urge to take in more food when more energy is needed, and the meaning of energy requirements. Your goal as an eater is to keep energy intake in balance. This way, you power your metabolism but avoid gaining weight.

Measuring Energy

Energy is the capacity to do work. A physicist would say energy is the ability to move matter against an opposing force. Picking up a bowling ball is work because you lift the ball even while gravity (an opposing force) tries to keep you from moving it. Cells perform work when they absorb nutrients. The cells must spend some energy because the membrane resists free passage for almost all nutrients except water.

Most people have a more difficult time estimating how much energy is in a particular food than estimating its nutrients. You probably could distinguish between the protein food and the carbohydrate food if a plate of steak and mashed potatoes were set before you. You most likely would also guess (correctly) that a salad of broccoli and carrots offers more vitamins than cotton candy! What about energy? Does a hamburger provide more or less energy than a hot dog? Does a bowl of chili energize better than a bowl of tomato soup?

Nutritionists solve the puzzle of energy in foods by putting food in a bomb calorimeter and measuring the amount of heat a food gives off when it's combusted. The food's heat value is then converted to either of two similar units of energy called the calorie and the kilojoule.

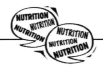

Nutrition Vocabulary

A calorie is the amount of heat that raises the temperature of 1 gram of water 1 degree Celsius. That's a fairly small amount of energy. Foods usually contain many calories, and the human body requires thousands of calories a day. To help simplify the math, nutritionists invented the kilocalorie, which equals 1,000 calories. In textbooks, a calorie is distinguished from a kilocalorie by capitalizing one. Thus, a regular calorie is *calorie* and a kilocalorie is *Calorie*, or, more commonly, a *kcal*.

Obviously, one poor typist could make that system collapse like a house of cards. Furthermore, nonscientists did not bother trying to tell calories apart from Calories. Nutritionists therefore decided that the word *calorie* would always mean a kilocalorie, regardless of whether it is capitalized or not. When you look up the calorie value of a food, you are probably really looking up its kilocalories.

Outside the United States and United Kingdom, nutritionists prefer using the kilojoule (kJ) to measure a unit of food energy. The comparison is 1 kJ equals about 0.24 calories (kilocalories); 1 calorie equals 4.2 kJ.

The Body's Energy Balance

The goal of eating is to supply enough energy and nutrients to maintain our metabolism. If we consume too much energy—too many calories—the body stores the extra energy in fat. If we take in too little energy—too few calories—the body must break down part of itself to supply the energy to run metabolism. The body starts with fats and carbohydrates, but in dire circumstances of low energy intake, it will degrade proteins for energy.

I assume you prefer not to become fat or emaciated. Instead, all of us would prefer to maintain a healthy energy balance. Energy balance in the body is simply the difference between how much energy is consumed and how much the body expends. Positive balance means intake is greater than expenditure, and negative balance occurs when expenditure exceeds intake:

➤ Energy intake > Energy output = Positive balance = Weight gain

➤ Energy intake < Energy output = Negative balance = Weight loss

Severe positive balance leads to obesity, and severe negative balance leads to starvation.

The body's energy balance is made up of three components:

1. Energy intake

2. Energy storage

3. Energy expenditure

You have some control over each of these components, so you can control your body's energy balance.

Energy Intake

Energy intake is the amount of energy contained in the foods you eat each day. Almost all foods are a blend, more or less, of carbohydrates, fats, and proteins. You will see in the next chapter that these foods supply different amounts of energy.

Energy Storage

When you eat a meal, your digestive tract digests the carbohydrates, fats, and proteins into smaller absorbable pieces. The cells lining the intestines absorb these substances and send them into the bloodstream, which carries them to all the cells of the body except for the cells that make up hair.

The body almost immediately uses the energy it needs to run basal metabolism, and then to power the activities that require additional energy. After these energy needs have been met, the body stores any excess energy.

Fat in adipose tissue is the major energy storage form. Fat is used for both short-term and long-term energy storage. The carbohydrate glycogen is more a short-term storage form for the body's energy and carbon. Protein also stores energy because amino acids can be used for energy if needed, but protein is always an energy source of last resort. The body uses protein for energy only in severe cases of starvation, when all fat and carbohydrate have been used up.

Nutrition Vocabulary

Adipose tissue serves as the main storage site of body fat. When no carbohydrates are available for energy, the body breaks down this tissue to generate energy.

Most adipose tissue lies beneath the deep layer of the skin called dermis. Adipose tissue is itself made up of cells called adipocytes of which there are two kinds. Adipocytes that make up white fat are involved in energy metabolism. White fat also insulates the body and forms protection for internal organs. These adipocytes are large and almost completely filled with a fat globule. Adipocytes that make up brown fat are more prevalent in babies and help produce heat for the newborn. These cells are smaller than white fat cells and contain smaller fat droplets.

Energy Expenditure

You can control energy intake by the amount and type of foods you eat. By decreasing the fat content of your diet, you automatically decrease energy intake. The types of foods in your diet also affect how you store energy. Diets higher in fats and carbohydrates lead to a higher amount of energy stored in adipose tissue and the liver (as glycogen).

To keep your body from storing too much energy, especially as adipose tissue—this is easy to monitor because you become overweight—you must expend energy. The best way to keep control over how much energy your body socks away in adipose is to balance expenditure with intake. The balance doesn't have to be perfect, but common sense should tell you that if you ingest extra calories, you will want to burn that excess by increasing energy expenditure. Otherwise, the excess calories get stored in adipose and your favorite jeans don't fit quite as well anymore.

Some energy in foods goes straight to supporting your basal metabolism. That's good because it is energy that you automatically use up so you don't stretch out your favorite jeans. Some energy then gets expended to digest a meal. This energy is called the thermic effect of a meal. This portion of energy intake is used to do the following:

➤ Digest food and absorb and transport nutrients

➤ Metabolize the food's nutrients

➤ Convert some of the nutrients in new cell constituents

➤ Store the new macromolecules you have made

Nutrition Morsels

Basal metabolism is the energy-demanding system that runs the involuntary actions in your body. These things are muscle contractions that control heartbeat, respiration, and digestive tract movement. Nutritionists speak of this energy requirement as the basal metabolic rate, or BMR. The BMR is the minimum level of energy your body must burn to sustain life in the awake state.

You cannot control basal metabolism or the thermic effect of meals. But there exists a third component of energy expenditure that you can control. It is physical activity.

Physical Activity

The best way to keep energy expenditure in line with intake is by adjusting the type and amount of physical activities you do. Nutritionists call the energy-burning feature of physical activity the thermic effect of exercise. We simply call it exercise. Exercise has three characteristics:

1. It involves the use of skeletal muscles for body movement.

2. It increases the body's metabolic rate.

3. It is the most variable aspect of energy metabolism, varying from day to day in the same person as well as varying between people.

To maintain energy balance, you strive to make sure all energy expenditures add up to your daily energy intake. Energy expenditure is the sum of three parts:

Energy expenditure = Basal metabolism + Thermic effect (meals) + Thermic effect (exercise)

Fortunately, you do not have to control all these intakes and outputs on your own. While you have the most control over what you put into your mouth (energy intake) and how you use some of those calories (physical activity), some automatic systems in the body help out.

How the Body Regulates Food Intake

The body helps you regulate your food intake. A combination of hormones, actions of the central nervous system, liver activity, and some external factors all work in concert to affect appetite, hunger, and satiety.

All three of these factors should be balanced in a way to prompt you to keep your food intake at an adequate level but also keep you from eating too much.

Appetite, Hunger, and Satiety

Appetite is the desire to eat. It is a component of your psychology the same as your urges to have sex, see a movie, or tell off that guy who just stole your parking space. Appetite usually relates to certain pleasant sensations you get from eating particular foods. Which affects your appetite more, an ice cream cone or a plate of chopped liver?

Hunger is a similar subjective feeling tied more to survival than to pleasure. Hunger can be distracting, nagging, or irritating to the point where most other activities seem less important. Hunger is a sensation that tells your body that finding a meal should be its highest priority.

Satiety is the opposite of hunger; it is a feeling of being well fed and not in need of another meal (for a while). Factors in the body that start the satiety sensation cause you to stop feeling hunger and (hopefully) terminate your eating.

Hunger and satiety are part of your body's physiology. When they work perfectly together, you maintain energy balance. Appetite, by contrast, is a learned response to food.

Factors Affecting Hunger

Five main factors work together to run your hunger-satiety sensations. Four of these factors are part of your physiology. The fifth factor comes from external situations that may be out of your control. For example, you may be hungry, but if food is not available at the moment, you cannot do anything about your hunger.

Let's first review the factors in the body that control hunger:

➤ Digestive tract: The presence of food or liquid in the stomach and small intestine causes some pressure that you feel as fullness. Certain substances on the cells lining the intestines detect carbohydrates and fats, and when this happens they cause your satiety response to increase. In addition, hormones are released during a meal, and they control feelings of hunger and satiety.

➤ Central nervous system: The hypothalamus section of the brain drives feelings of hunger and thirst and controls the part of the nervous system that regulates food intake.

➤ Circulatory system: After digesting a meal and absorbing nutrients, the levels of glucose, amino acids, fats, and other substances increase in the blood. The metabolic rate of the liver begins to increase as these substances arrive. This response by the liver may play a part in regulating food intake. When the levels of nutrients in the blood fall below a certain threshold several hours after a meal, the hunger response again begins to build.

➤ Adipose tissue: Fat cells produce the hormone leptin, which communicates directly with the hypothalamus on matters related to hunger and food intake.

Nutrition Morsels

Adiposity signals are sent out by three hormones to your brain to communicate the levels of stored energy in your adipose tissue. As long as fat stores are adequate, the hormones leptin, insulin, and adiponectin tell the hypothalamus that all is well and there is no need to turn on the hunger response.

External Factors Affecting Food Intake

Some external factors affect food intake and even hunger. The appearance, odor, taste, and presentation of food have a big impact on your response to food. Pretend you are a person who loves steak. Which is more appealing to you: a steak cooked medium-rare and still sizzling from the grill or a conveyer belt loaded with cuts of meat fresh from a slaughterhouse?

Perhaps color affects your response to a food. Which appeals more: mashed potatoes whipped creamy white or a similar serving turned blue with food coloring?

Finally, nutritionists also realize that much more serious psychological factors affect a person's response to food, appetite, and perhaps even hunger. Depression is known to increase or decrease food intake in certain people, or change the type of foods a person wants.

Other factors that may affect appetite and hunger are time of day, peer pressure, anxiety, and cultural preferences.

Physical Activity and Hunger

When ingested food is needed for physical activities, you convert the chemical energy of the food into mechanical energy of movement. This involves a series of interconnected reactions in the body. The carbohydrates and fats first get broken down, and then their breakdown products go into the series of reactions that make up respiration.

Respiration cranks out more and more ATPs to drive the energy-demanding process of contracting muscle. Those contractions add up to a simple movement such as turning your eyes to spot a tennis ball or running toward the ball, readying your racket, and swinging the racket to return the ball over the net. Hundreds of muscles gobble up millions of ATP molecules for that single return. Let's hope it's a winner!

Hunger increases with increased physical activity, but the increase is not proportional. If you normally do very little exercise, you will notice your appetite increase if you begin riding a bicycle for an hour each day. Hunger might increase even more if you decided to train six days a week for a triathlon. But would hunger go out of control if you signed up for Marine Corps boot camp and exerted yourself for almost three weeks with little rest? Hunger is only one component of your body's physiology and energy requirements.

Your body adjusts a bit over time to operate more efficiently in sustained physical activity. Thus, the body does not burn calories the exact same way in your first-ever mile run compared with 1 mile of running that is part of your daily training for a marathon. The nervous and circulatory systems, your musculature, and bones all adjust to increased physical activity. Though your appetite will certainly increase with increased exercise, so will your efficiency in using, metabolizing, and storing nutrients and energy.

Nutrition Morsels

Nutritionists divide people into two general groups based on energy balance and typical levels of daily physical activity: sedentary and physically active. A sedentary person does zero or near zero minutes a day engaged in exercise that raises the heart rate. An active person engages in about 60 minutes a day of exercise. By comparing the ratio of these individuals' resting metabolic rate to energy expenditure, scientists show that active people are more efficient at using the energy from food than are sedentary people.

Energy Requirements

Energy requirements vary from person to person. The main factors that determine your daily energy needs are age, gender, and level of physical activity:

➤ Children, 2–3 years: 1,000 kcal sedentary (S); 1,400 kcal active (A)

➤ Females, 4–8 years: 1,200 kcal (S); 1,800 kcal (A)

➤ Females, 9–13 years: 1,600 kcal (S); 2,200 kcal (A)

➤ Females, 14–18 years: 1,800 kcal (S); 2,400 kcal (A)

➤ Females, 19–30 years: 2,000 kcal (S); 2,400 kcal (A)

➤ Females, 31–50 years: 1,800 kcal (S); 2,200 kcal (A)

➤ Females, 51+ years: 1,600 kcal (S); 2,200 kcal (A)

➤ Males, 4–8 years: 1,200 kcal (S); 2,000 kcal (A)

➤ Males, 9–13 years: 1,800 kcal (S); 2,600 kcal (A)

➤ Males, 14–18 years: 2,200 kcal (S); 3,200 kcal (A)

➤ Males, 19–30 years: 2,400 kcal (S); 3,000 kcal (A)

➤ Males, 31–50 years: 2,200 kcal (S); 3,000 kcal (A)

➤ Males, 51+ years: 2,000 kcal (S); 2,800 kcal (A)

Depending on your average level of physical activity per day, your energy requirement falls somewhere inside these ranges for sedentary and very active people.

CHAPTER 7

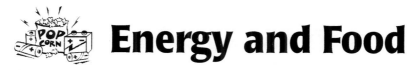

Energy and Food

In This Chapter

- ➤ Energy pyramids and you
- ➤ Where our food energy originates
- ➤ How to calculate your food's calories
- ➤ Is breakfast really the most important meal?

In this chapter I explain how food carries energy from the Sun to you. Humans are one small part of a massive flow of energy on Earth, from the nonliving solar system to every living thing. This chapter explains nutrition in the big picture. You will learn about food chains and food webs and how they, and you, fit into something called the energy pyramid.

This chapter also explains why different foods supply you with different amounts of energy. You will learn about nutrient density and energy density of foods. By understanding these terms, you'll be able to make better choices, opting for foods that will energize you for hours and deliver other essential nutrients. Put another way, you will learn why selecting a chicken salad for lunch is better than selecting a candy bar.

The Energy Pyramid

All living things on Earth are connected by how they use and share energy. Energy comes to Earth in a one-way direction from the Sun. Photosynthetic organisms are the only living things that can capture that solar energy. These organisms are green plants, algae, and photosynthetic bacteria.

Photosynthetic organisms use the energy to run their metabolism, but in so doing they also serve all other living things. By capturing solar energy and storing it as chemical energy, photosynthetic organisms produce our energy source for life. For this reason, biologists call photosynthetic organisms producers. Every animal that cannot run photosynthesis must get energy by consuming the producers or by eating an animal that eats producers. Thus, humans and other animal life are called consumers.

The flow of energy from producers to consumers moves in one direction. Picture millions of tiny photosynthetic organisms creating the foundation of this energy flow. A smaller yet still enormous number of small organisms feed on these photosynthetic producers. In turn, larger animals feed on the tiny organisms. Larger animals yet prey on the smaller ones. As you look at this flow of energy from prey to predator, you might notice two features:

1. The number of predators is usually less than the number of prey animals.

2. The body size of predators is usually larger than that of their prey.

This flow of energy and food describes a food chain. Most food chains begin with producers and end with a predator said to be at the top of its food chain. Examples of animals at the top of the food chain are eagles, owls, lions, sharks, grizzly bears, and humans.

Each food chain also has animals that live in the intermediate levels. In these intermediate levels, an animal that is a predator often becomes prey for another predator. Thus, a fox might snatch a hare one evening, then get eaten by a bobcat the following night.

Because the numbers of producers are enormous and the numbers of organisms at each successive level decrease, this energy flow is pictured in the shape of a pyramid.

Energy pyramids have two characteristics that impact the health of humans, who sit atop their food chain:

➤ Moving up the food chain from each level to the next, some energy is lost and cannot be recovered by a predator. This energy goes into the environment as heat. So as energy moves up a food chain from producers to final consumers, the efficiency of getting energy and nutrients from one level to the next decreases. Being at the top of a food chain or energy pyramid may sound great, but it is actually a very inefficient way to survive.

➤ While energy gets lost moving up a food chain, many chemicals become more and more concentrated. Turnover rates of chemicals that hide in fat or bone are not quick. When a predator eats a prey animal, these chemicals become even more concentrated in the predator's tissue. For most nutrients this may be only a minor concern because the body eventually uses up the nutrient, even fat soluble nutrients. But dangerous chemicals in foods can accumulate in a food chain until the top predator gets an almost lethal dose. This accumulation of chemicals from organisms at the bottom of a food chain to the top is called bioaccumulation.

Nutrition Vocabulary

Turnover rate refers to how fast a chemical in your body or in nature gets replaced. In nutrition, fast turnover means that a nutrient is being used up faster than it can be replaced. Slow turnover means that a nutrient does not get used up quickly and may even accumulate in the body. Turnover rates of nutrients are usually relative to each other. Therefore, proteins have a much slower turnover rate than most B vitamins.

Herbivores, Carnivores, and Omnivores

Producers make their own chemicals for building new cells by capturing the Sun's energy and getting carbon from carbon dioxide in the atmosphere. Consumers can only get energy and nutrients by eating producers or each other!

As consumers evolved on Earth, they branched out into three types of animals based on the main foods that make up their diet:

> ➤ Herbivores: Eat only plants and have teeth designed to harvest and grind plant fibers and a digestive tract designed to ferment plant fibers and get energy from them.

> ➤ Carnivores: Eat only other animals and have teeth designed to cut animal tissue. Carnivores get some plant nutrients from the partially digested foods in the digestive tract of their prey.

> ➤ Omnivores: Eat both plant and animal tissue and have teeth designed for both types of food as well as a digestive tract designed to digest and absorb all nutrients except fiber. Examples are humans and bears.

The Energy Value of Protein, Carbohydrates, and Fats

While you sit smugly atop your food chain, where do you get most of your energy? Since humans are omnivores, we get energy and nutrients from plant and animal foods. The main sources of energy are carbohydrates, fats, and proteins. Vitamins and minerals do not supply energy directly, but they are essential for getting energy out of carbohydrates, fats, and proteins.

These three nutrients contain the following calories (kcal) per gram (g):

➤ Carbohydrates: 4 kcal/g

➤ Fats: 9 kcal/g

➤ Proteins: 4 kcal/g

Very few foods are 100 percent carbohydrate, fat, or protein. Our diet is made up of foods that provide all three plus water, fiber, vitamins, and minerals in widely varying amounts. To devise a healthy diet, you want to:

Nutrition Morsels

Does alcohol have any nutritional value? Alcohol gives the body some energy. One gram of alcohol supplies about 7 kcal of energy.

1. Maximize the nutrients and energy you get from food.

2. Include many of your favorite foods.

3. Balance your energy intake and expenditure so that you do not gain too much or lose too much weight, assuming you are already at an ideal weight for your age and height.

To accomplish these objectives, it helps to know a bit about nutrient density and energy density of foods.

You can find easy-to-use online energy calculators at www.myfoodrecord.com and http://calorielab.com.

Calculating Calories

Anyone can estimate the number of kcal they ingest using the 4-9-4 method. This method is based on the approximate kcal of energy in carbohydrates, fats, and proteins, respectively. First, look at a food's packaging to find out how many grams of carbohydrate, fat, and protein you get with each serving.

For example, a hamburger with lettuce on a bun might contain 40 grams of carbohydrate, 32 grams of fat, and 35 grams of protein. To calculate the kcal of energy from each nutrient, you would multiply by the kcal per gram values:

➤ Carbohydrates = 40 × 4 = 160 kcal

➤ Fats = 32 × 9 = 288 kcal

➤ Proteins = 35 × 4 = 140 kcal

Your hamburger adds up to 588 kcal. Notice that almost 50 percent of the kcal comes from fat.

Nutrient Density and Energy Density

Nutrient density of a food is an indication of its quality. Nutritionists determine a food's nutrient density by comparing the amount of protein, vitamins, or minerals it offers to the amount of calories it carries. A nutrient-dense food is one that provides a high amount of one or more nutrients with a relatively small amount of calories.

Examples of nutrient-dense foods are:

➤ Lean meats

➤ Low-fat or fat-free milk

➤ Beans

➤ Broccoli

➤ Whole-wheat bread

➤ Whole-grain cereals

The opposite of nutrient-dense foods are empty-calorie foods. These are foods that are high in carbohydrates, sugar, or fats but provide very few other nutrients.

Nutrition Morsels

Empty calories come from foods that provide few nutrients yet carry a large number of calories. Cookies, cake, potato chips, and soft drinks are the best examples of empty-calorie foods.

Compare a 12-ounce can of soft drink with the same serving of fat-free milk. The soft drink contains about 37 grams of carbohydrate, all in the form of sugar, plus 35 milligrams or so of sodium. Those may be the only two nutrients the soft drink provides while also dumping 140 calories into your body. The 12-ounce glass of milk has about half the calories, and it delivers significant amounts of calcium, protein, and vitamins A and C, as well as several B vitamins.

Energy density works in a somewhat opposite manner to nutrient density. An energy-dense food is one that is high in calories, but the food itself weighs relatively little. Examples of energy-dense foods are:

➤ Cookies

➤ Nuts

➤ Butter

➤ Bacon

➤ Peanut butter

➤ Most fried foods, including potato chips and tortilla chips

Eating foods of low energy density help you feel full faster, yet they do not pack in a lot of calories. Therefore, you adjust your energy balance by incorporating more of these low-energy-density foods in your diet:

➤ Fruits

➤ Vegetables

➤ Spaghetti

➤ Baked potato (without toppings!)

➤ Cooked rice

➤ Cottage cheese

➤ Breakfast cereals, including oatmeal

The Best Way to Energize Yourself

Swearing off potato chips and soft drinks forever might not be necessary to achieve good nutrition. You may have noticed by now that good nutrition is built on balance. By this I mean a balance of food groups, nutrients, and energy sources. With a balanced diet, a healthy person can enjoy an occasional treat such as ice cream, birthday cake, or a beer and still have a sound overall nutrition plan.

What are the best ways to improve your energy balance and still enjoy the foods you eat? The following tips provide good direction for setting you on the correct path to good nutrition. Are there other ways to achieve a healthy nutrition plan? Of course. But these tips are consistently mentioned by nutrition experts as the best ways to improve your nutrition and energy balance:

➤ Exercise: Physical activity makes the body use energy and nutrients more efficiently, and it burns fat.

➤ Eat a variety of foods: Selecting foods from grains, vegetables, fruits, meat, beans, dairy products, and oils each day is the easiest way to ensure you are getting a balanced intake of nutrients and energy. These food groups will be discussed in more detail in later chapters.

➤ Pay attention to nutrient density and energy density: Don't obsess, but try to think about these two qualities of food at every meal.

➤ Eat breakfast: This meal gives you the energy and nutrients you need after a period of fasting for ten hours or more. Do your best to select foods from as many food groups as possible.

➤ Choose carbohydrates wisely: Carbohydrates are your body's main source of energy and a necessary nutrient. The type of carbohydrate you choose, however, makes a great difference in energy metabolism. Sugars are fast-burning carbohydrates. Some sugar in the diet is okay, but try to balance sugars with carbohydrates that release their energy more slowly. These slow-burning carbohydrates are called complex carbohydrates and include starches and fibers.

➤ Know your fats: Later in this book you will be introduced to the good fats and the bad fats. As a rule of thumb, look at fats this way: polyunsaturated fats are good and saturated and trans fats are bad. Good fats are found in olive oil, canola oil, nuts, and avocados. Bad fats show up in red meats, butter, lard, and prepared foods such as custards and icings.

➤ Think protein first, then carbohydrates and fats: Energy balance comes mainly from carbohydrates and fats, but proteins rule the body in the form of enzymes. View every meal and snack based on the proteins they contain relative to the sugars and bad fats.

➤ Drink water: Water is the material in which all your chemical reactions take place. Your energy-generating reactions simply cannot work if you are dehydrated. Adult women should get about eleven cups of water each day and men need about sixteen cups. Remember that some of this water can come from fruits, vegetables, soups, and beverages.

➤ Adjust your meal frequency: Not everyone must stick to the three square meals a day approach, and in fact this may not work best for your particular body metabolism. If you've followed all the tips above and cannot get that energy boost you feel you should be getting from food, try several smaller meals throughout the day rather than the traditional "three squares." Our ancestors probably didn't evolve by sticking to a strict breakfast-lunch-dinner schedule.

➤ Limit coffee: If you're like me, you have tried skipping a few of the tips above by substituting a strong cup of coffee. The chemical caffeine in coffee stimulates certain nerve functions that fool you into thinking you have more energy. Coffee can make the heart beat faster, increases respiration rate, and gives you a sense of alertness. Coffee also increases dehydration, and its benefits wear off in about two hours in most people. Coffee is neither a nutrient nor a food group. Nevertheless, I do not believe coffee represents the demise of good nutrition. One or two cups a day, switching to decaffeinated coffee, or substituting tea, especially herbal teas, are reasonable approaches to managing your coffee intake.

Is Breakfast the Most Important Meal?

Exercise guru Jack LaLanne used to say, "Eat breakfast like a king, lunch like a prince, and dinner like a pauper." His point was clear: breakfast is an important meal. Is it the most important meal? Consider what happens to lots of adults and children who skip breakfast:

➤ Tiredness increases and alertness and concentration decrease by mid-morning.

➤ The urge to snack increases and those snacks are often caffeinated or high-sugar foods that make you feel like you've gotten a burst of energy.

➤ A habit of skipping breakfast has been correlated in scientific studies with heart disease, diabetes, and obesity.

The American Dietetic Association stresses that breakfasts can include whatever foods you want as long as they are good nutrient-dense sources of carbohydrates for energy and protein for endurance. I've listed here some traditional, as well as some less traditional, breakfasts that fill these requirements:

➤ Low-sugar cereal with fruit and yogurt

➤ Oatmeal with raisins and nuts

➤ Whole-grain toast with peanut butter and fruit

➤ Hard-boiled egg sliced into a whole-grain pita

➤ Scrambled eggs, turkey bacon, and fruit

➤ Chicken noodle, vegetable, or bean soup

➤ Chicken burrito

➤ Peanut butter and jelly sandwich on whole-grain bread

➤ Beef chili with cheese

➤ Turkey, tomato, and avocado sandwich on whole-grain bread.

Nutrition Morsels

Caffeine is a nitrogen-containing chemical that inhibits an enzyme involved in ATP metabolism. With this enzyme inhibited, the body starts accumulating a chemical called cyclic AMP or c-AMP for short. As c-AMP levels rise, the body is stimulated to keep glucose circulating in the bloodstream rather than store it. Cells continue to absorb the glucose and burn it for energy even if the body does not necessarily need this extra energy. Eventually, the caffeine effect on c-AMP subsides and you get a feeling of crashing. Caffeine gives you a temporary jolt of energy because it short circuits the normal energy-generating reactions in your cells.

PART THREE

Starches, Fats, and Proteins

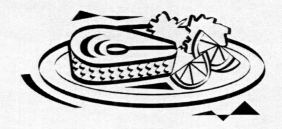

CHAPTER 8

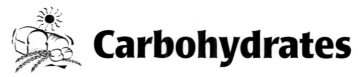 **Carbohydrates**

In This Chapter

➤ The job of carbohydrates

➤ The main simple and complex carbohydrates in food

➤ How the body uses carbohydrates

➤ How the body digests, absorbs, and stores carbohydrates

In this chapter you meet the carbohydrates. Carbohydrates have gone into and out of favor in nutrition over the past several decades. About four decades ago, Americans began learning that too much red meat in their diet might be associated with heart problems and other health issues. They turned to pasta, rice, and breads. The carbohydrates in these foods seemed to represent a "clean" nutrient that would not clog arteries or stretch the waistline. But today carbohydrates are vilified as the main cause of our obesity problem. Among carbohydrates, perhaps nothing has received more blame than sugar.

This chapter presents the truth about carbohydrates. Simply, carbohydrates are nutrients. By that definition alone you know that your body needs carbohydrates at certain levels in your daily diet for balanced nutrition and good health. Pay attention here: carbohydrates are good for you.

Where people run into trouble regarding carbohydrates occurs when the diet becomes unbalanced. Taking in too many carbohydrates in relation to fat and protein causes trouble. This imbalance is true for any nutrient, not just carbs.

This chapter covers all things carbohydrate. It describes what carbohydrates do in the body, how the body digests and uses them, and the main types of carbohydrates likely to make up a large portion of the American diet.

What Carbohydrates Do in the Body

Carbohydrates make up only about 3 percent of your cells, but there are more than two hundred different carbohydrates that play important roles in metabolism.

The two major roles of carbohydrate in the body are as the main energy sources for metabolism and the main source of carbon for body chemistry. In addition to these two big jobs, carbohydrates also do the following:

➤ Store carbon and energy in the form of glycogen

➤ Make up part of the substances on the outer surface of cells that help cells communicate with each other

➤ Participate in the immune system activity in fighting infection

➤ Make up part of the physical structure of cells and act as part of the body's structural framework

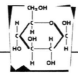

The Chemistry of Nutrition

Carbon is useful in Earth chemistry because a carbon atom has the ability to attach to four other chemicals at the same time. This is a rare quality for most elements of the body. Carbon atoms also have the ability to connect into long chains that are either straight or branched into side chains.

One of Earth's simplest carbon chemicals is the gas carbon dioxide (CO_2). Carbon dioxide is essential for photosynthesis. From carbon dioxide, photosynthetic organisms make the other organic compounds that other living things need to live.

Carbohydrates in the form of sugars also combine with proteins or lipids to make substances with specialized roles in nerve function, immunity, and cell structure. When a sugar attaches to a protein it forms a glycoprotein. When it attaches to a fat or fatlike compound, it forms a glycolipid.

Types of Carbohydrates

Photosynthesis produces all the carbohydrates, directly or indirectly, that's needed for life. In photosynthesis, carbon dioxide gas is used as a building block for making the sugar glucose:

$$6\ CO_2 + 2\ H_2O \rightarrow C_6H_{12}O_6 + 6\ O_2$$

You can see how important photosynthesis is to us; it is a source of oxygen (O_2) in the atmosphere as well as a source of our main energy carbohydrate. Photosynthetic and non-photosynthetic organisms collectively produce all the other organic compounds that define life on Earth.

Chemists divide carbohydrates into two major groups: simple and complex. Simple carbohydrates are mainly sugars. Sugars have a basic chemical structure of CH_2O, such as glucose, which has six carbons to make the formula shown in the above equation. Complex carbohydrates are structures larger than sugars. They contain many sugars connected to each other. The two main types of complex carbohydrates in your diet are starches and fibers.

Simple Carbohydrates

Simple carbohydrates consist of monosaccharides and disaccharides. Monosaccharides contain only one unit of sugar, which makes up the entire chemical structure. Disaccharides contain two sugar units linked together. The sugars in disaccharides can either be the same or different sugars.

The monosaccharides common in our diet are usually trioses (containing three carbon atoms), tetroses, (containing four carbons), pentoses (five carbons), or hexoses (six carbons):

➤ Trioses ($C_3H_6O_3$): Glyceraldehyde and dihydroxyacetone

➤ Tetroses ($C_4H_8O_4$): Erythrose

➤ Pentoses ($C_5H_{10}O_5$): Ribose, arabinose, xylose, and xylulose

➤ Hexoses ($C_6H_{12}O_6$): Glucose, galactose, mannose, and fructose

Common disaccharides are:

➤ Sucrose ($C_{12}H_{22}O_{11}$): Glucose and fructose

➤ Maltose ($C_{12}H_{22}O_{11}$): Glucose and glucose

➤ Cellobiose ($C_{12}H_{22}O_{11}$): Glucose and glucose

➤ Lactose ($C_{12}H_{22}O_{11}$): Glucose and Galactose

Notice that the disaccharides shown here have the same chemical formula and maltose and cellobiose are both disaccharides made of two glucoses. Why then are they all not the same thing? Maltose and cellobiose differ by how the two glucoses link to each other. Chemists say that maltose contains an alpha (α) linkage between glucoses and cellobiose contains a beta (β) linkage. Digestive enzymes secreted by the human gut are much better at cleaving alpha linkages than they are at breaking apart beta linkages. Thus, you digest the disaccharide maltose better than you digest cellobiose.

Complex Carbohydrates

Complex carbohydrates are long chains of sugars linked together. Very long chains of sugars are called polysaccharides and relatively short chains are called oligosaccharides. Nutritionists also include fibers with complex carbohydrates even though some fibers bear little resemblance to the true carbohydrates such as starch. (Fibers perhaps get lumped in with complex carbohydrates because they all come from plants.)

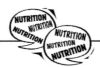

Nutrition Vocabulary

You may occasionally see the term *oligosaccharides* in reference to complex carbohydrates. Some nutritionists prefer to use this term for carbohydrates made of two to six sugars. Therefore, a disaccharide would be classified as an oligosaccharide. Other oligosaccharides would be trisaccharides (three sugars), tetrasaccharides (four sugars), pentasaccharides (five sugars), and hexasaccharides (six sugars).

A common trisaccharide is raffinose, composed of glucose, fructose, and galactose. A common tetrasaccharide is stachyose, which contains an extra galactose. Both oligosaccharides are found in a variety of vegetables such as broccoli, cabbage, and brussels sprouts.

Like disaccharides, complex carbohydrates can be composed of all the same sugar or different sugars. The main complex carbohydrates likely to be in your diet are polysaccharides. Their digestibility and percentage of your diet varies. For example, the polysaccharide starch is very common in American diets and often makes up a high percentage of a meal. Think about how much starch you ingest when you eat a baked potato. By contrast, some polysaccharides are relatively rare in the American diet. For example, chitin is found mainly in the shell of shellfish or insects. How often do you think you ingest chitin?

The amount of polysaccharide in the human diet is roughly proportional to our ability to digest it. For instance, we have no trouble digesting starch, but the human digestive cannot digest chitin.

The main polysaccharides in our diet are listed below in order of prevalence and digestibility. I put a star next to the ones that are often also classified as fibers because we digest them poorly or not at all.

➤ Starch: The most digestible polysaccharide; made of repeating glucose units. This nutrient is a major energy source in the human diet and in the diet of many animals and microbes as well.

➤ Dextrins: Polysaccharides that result from a partial breakdown of starch in nature. Seeds and plants that have been heated or dried might hold high amounts of dextrins compared with starches.

➤ Glycogen: The polysaccharide of animal origin, found mainly in the liver and in muscle. It is composed of only glucose units but has different chemical linkages and branching patterns than starch.

➤ Cellulose*: Humans and animals with similar digestive tracts (pigs, dogs, and cats) have a hard time digesting this polysaccharide. It is made of many glucose units strung together in linkages that our enzymes do not easily degrade.

➤ Hemicellulose*: This is a heterogeneous mixture of at least five different sugars linked together in strands and branches. In plants, a variety of hemicelluloses strengthens the plant stalk and stem.

➤ Pectin*: This polysaccharide resides between the cells of plants. It both strengthens the plant and holds the plant's cells together. When a plant is either heated up or chilled, you can extract the pectin as a gel-like material. Any jelly expert will tell you that pectin is the stuff that makes fruit juices solidify into jelly and jam.

➤ Gums: These polysaccharides from plants help plants heal injuries by forming a thick fluid. People take advantage of this quality by using plant gums as thickeners in many food and nonfood products. Most gums contain long chains of mainly the sugars glucuronic acid and galacturonic acid.

➤ Mucilages: These heterogeneous polysaccharides are found mainly in seeds, bark, and seaweed. They contain mostly galactose and mannose with a variety of other sugars.

➤ Mucopolysaccharides: Another group of polysaccharides of animal origin, these substances make up a large part of animal connective tissue, such as cartilage.

➤ Chitin: This almost indestructible material is made of the sugar-like chemical acetyl-glucosamine. Chitin strengthens the outer skeleton (exoskeleton), or shell, of insects and crustaceans. Very few organisms in nature can degrade this material. Certain fungi secrete the enzyme chitinase, which breaks down chitin and prevents it from building up in nature.

Nutrition Morsels

Humans can easily digest two types of starch that are both common in our diets. These starches are amylose and amylopectin. Amylose is made of mainly long, straight chains of glucose. Amylopectin also contains chains of glucose, but they branch off into numerous side chains. Amylose makes up about 20 percent of our dietary starches; amylopectin makes up 80 percent.

Nutrition Morsels

Lactose is the main carbohydrate in milk. This disaccharide is degraded by the enzyme lactase in the small intestine to the sugars glucose and galactose. As infants, we depend on lactose as an important energy source in our diet. As we get older, lactose becomes less important in supplying energy and other carbohydrates give ample amounts of glucose to keep metabolism running. With age, as much as 75 percent of the population loses lactase activity.

With lowered lactase activity, much of the lactose in dairy products escapes from the small intestine to the large intestine. There, bacteria see the lactose as a bounty of easily digestible energy. These bacteria gobble up the lactose and rapidly ferment it. The fermentations produce large amounts of microbial end products, including gases. Although your bacteria may be deliriously happy to see lactose coming their way, your experience is quite different. The inability to digest lactose is called lactose intolerance. You are likely to experience abdominal cramping, gas, and possibly diarrhea.

How We Digest Carbohydrates

Starch digestion begins in the mouth where the enzyme salivary amylase breaks down part of this nutrient. The rest of the digestion and absorption of simple carbohydrates and polysaccharides takes place in the small intestine. After digestive enzymes have broken apart the carbohydrates into single sugars, the cells lining the small intestine absorb the sugars and send them into the bloodstream.

Large polysaccharides and fibers are digested wholly or partially in the large intestine. Most of the enzymes that do this work come from an immense population of bacteria that normally live in your large intestine. Bacterial enzymes liberate additional sugars from the complex carbohydrates that made it through the mouth, stomach, and small intestine mostly undigested.

The digestive tract absorbs only single sugars. So you must be able to digest disaccharides and larger carbohydrates to this basic unit before they can do you any good. The cells lining your intestines are best at absorbing glucose, galactose, and fructose. This works out well since these are also among the most common sugars in food. The portal vein then transports these sugars to the liver where galactose and fructose are largely removed. After blood passes through the liver, the main sugar remaining in blood circulating to the rest of the body is glucose.

The Enzymes that Digest Carbohydrates

You may have noticed by now that many enzymes end with the suffix *ase*. Proteins are digested by proteases, lipids are digested by lipases, and carbohydrates are digested by a raft of other *ases*. The carbohydrate-digesting enzymes made by you or your bacteria are:

➤ Amylase: Degrades starches

➤ Sucrase: Digests sucrose

➤ Maltase: Digests maltose

➤ Lactase: Digests lactose

➤ Cellobiase: Made by bacteria to digest cellobiose

➤ Cellulase: Made by bacteria to digest cellulose

How We Store Carbohydrates

Plants store energy mainly as starch; animals store energy mainly as glycogen. Glycogen looks a lot like amylopectin. It contains strings of glucoses linked together with extensive side branches.

As glucose enters the liver, hormones control whether the liver should ship the glucose right out into the bloodstream or save it for later. When glucose levels in the blood are already high, the hormone insulin also increases. Insulin then prompts the liver to store the glucose. An enzyme called glycogen synthase starts to add glucoses onto existing stores of glycogen, like adding new beads to a strand of beads.

If your body begins to need more energy and blood glucose levels are low, the hormone glucagon steps into action. Glucagon induces an enzyme

Nutrition Morsels

Carbo-loading is a process in which a person ingests a large proportion of dietary carbohydrates for about six days before an athletic event. The process also involves decreased exercise, called tapering, so that the liver stores all the excess glucose and does not burn it until it is needed. Carbo-loading can increase a person's glycogen levels by more than 50 percent above normal, but many nutritionists question whether it helps with overall athletic performance.

(glucosidase) to start breaking glucoses off of the glycogen molecule. These glucoses enter the bloodstream and circulate to the hungry cells that need them.

Nutrition Morsels

Diabetes is the name for several diseases involving abnormal carbohydrate metabolism. Discussions of diabetes usually refer to diabetes mellitus, a chronic condition of hyperglycemia or excess glucose in the blood. This comes from either a failure of the pancreas to produce enough of the hormone insulin (type 1 diabetes mellitus) or insulin resistance by the body's cells (type 2 diabetes mellitus). Both types can be treated with special diets and medications.

How We Use Carbohydrates for Energy

Glucose is the major energy source for all animals. Our cells take in glucose and use its carbon to make new carbohydrates, proteins, and fats. As cells break down glucose, they also recover the energy that the sugar holds in its chemical bonds.

The body gets energy from glucose by feeding it to a series of enzymes that make up a process called glycolysis. The term *lysis* refers to something being broken apart. In glycolysis, a glucose molecule is literally broken apart. Glycolysis forms two new products each of which contain three carbons.

The products of glycolysis then enter a new set of reactions that are part of respiration. Glycolysis gives us a little bit of energy in the form of the compound ATP. Most of our energy, however, comes from respiration. Glycolysis produces about two ATPs every time it breaks down one glucose. Respiration produces more than thirty ATPs every time it runs.

Can We Make Glucose?

The body can produce its own glucose in dire circumstances. For instance, if you were to fast for more than about twenty hours, the enzymes of glycolysis begin to run in reverse. Instead of breaking down glucose, these enzymes take the compound lactate and begin to assemble glucose from it in the liver. This process is called gluconeogenesis or the Cori cycle.

You cannot survive with gluconeogenesis alone; sooner or later you need food to give you more glucose. But for a short period, gluconeogenesis helps feed starving cells the carbon and energy they need.

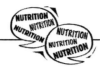

Nutrition Vocabulary

Lactate, or lactic acid, is a chemical made of three carbons and produced by muscle cells. It builds up in muscle during extreme exertion when the body's need for ATP exceeds the ability to take in enough oxygen. In other words, respiration can't run fast enough to meet the cells' energy demands. In this situation, the end products of glycolysis begin to build up and much of the end products get turned into lactate. Lactate buildup after intense exercise can be felt as soreness in certain overworked muscles.

After the exertion ends, lactate circulates to the liver, where it slowly gets converted back to glucose via the gluconeogenesis pathway.

CHAPTER 9

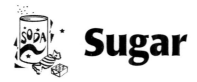 **Sugar**

In This Chapter

➤ The types and amount of sugars in food

➤ Sweeteners and sweetener scores

➤ Slow sugars, fast sugars, and the glycemic index

In this chapter you become better acquainted with the good and the bad of sugar.

Without sugar, your metabolism stops. Glycolysis runs only when fed a steady input of glucose, a sugar. Your cells cannot divide and reproduce without DNA, and DNA is built on a backbone of ribose, another sugar. Your cells communicate with each other because of the sugars attached to their surfaces. Your immune system protects you against infection because of the sugars that make up its components.

Perhaps humans evolved with a particular craving for sugar because it's so critical for life. Sugar certainly tempts us. Early humans probably followed their craving for sugar when heading out to hunt and gather the foods that made up their diet. But who the heck is out there hunting and gathering these days? Why do respected scientists now call sugar a toxin or a poison or even evil?

Remember my stressing the importance of a balanced diet? One way to undermine good nutrition is by eating too much of one type of food while ignoring other essential nutrients. That has happened with many of us and the relationship we have with sugar.

Sugar in Food

You need sugar. You also probably get too much sugar because of two things that makes sugar useful to food manufacturers: sugar is sweet and most people are attracted to sweet foods, and sugar is an excellent preservative. For these two reasons, the food industry adds sugar to many processed foods to enhance their palatability and to keep the food from spoiling.

Nutrition Morsels

Sugar works as an effective food preservative because it chemically binds to water molecules. (Salt works as a preservative the same way.) When water becomes bound to sugar, it simultaneously becomes unavailable for biological reactions. Microbes such as bacteria, molds, and yeasts need water to grow. If lots of sugar has tied up all the water in a food, these microbes cannot grow and therefore cannot ruin the food.

Certain foods are bountiful sources of ready-to-use energy. In other words, these are foods that supply you with a lot of sugar and few other nutrients. Nutritionists refer to these foods as having a high percentage of calories from carbohydrates:

➤ Table sugar, sometimes called saccharose: Made up entirely of sucrose.

➤ Honey: A sucrose that has been partially broken down into glucose and fructose. It also contains a small amount of a variety of other disaccharides, oligosaccharides, and some amino acids.

➤ Jelly and jam: Contain a variety of sugars and disaccharides, mainly glucose, fructose, and sucrose.

➤ Fruit: Contains large amounts a fructose but is also a good source of other carbohydrates and fiber.

➤ Potato: Contains large amounts of starch made up entirely of thousands of glucoses.

All of these foods deliver a large amount of glucose with each bite. Your body doesn't care whether the glucose comes from a shaker, a beehive, or a baked potato—it all gets used the same way by cells, namely, in glycolysis.

Other foods that yield a lot of sugar contain about 75 percent of all their calories in the form of easily digestible starches. These are corn, rice, breads, corn flakes, and noodles. Again, the body does not care where it gets glucose as long as it gets enough to energize all your vital systems.

Fast Sugar versus Slow Sugar

The main difference between sugar foods and starchy foods is the speed of getting glucose into your bloodstream. The body can digest high-sugar foods such as honey, candy, and soda very quickly, so the body gets a big influx of sugar all at once. Large sugar-containing substances, such as polysaccharides, take longer to digest. As a result, their glucose units are released more slowly and get absorbed into the bloodstream more evenly.

Types of Food Sugars

The main sugars found naturally in foods are glucose and fructose. Fructose is sometimes called fruit sugar because it occurs in high amounts in fruits but it is also abundant in many vegetables and in honey.

The disaccharides maltose and lactose also supply sugars to you after digestive enzymes break them down into two glucoses (maltose) or a glucose and a galactose (lactose). The body converts fructose and galactose into chemicals that can enter glycolysis just like glucose can. Thus, all three of these sugars serve as good energy sources.

Oligosaccharides and polysaccharides, such as starch, also supply the body with ample amounts of glucose that go either into glycolysis for energy or glycogen for storage.

Nutrition Morsels

Maltose and lactose are disaccharides that supply the body with glucose, but they come from very different sources. Maltose is malt sugar and is one of the least common disaccharides in nature. It is present in many seeds during the germinating (sprouting) stage.

Lactose is the milk sugar produced by mammals. Lactose makes up 4–6 percent of cow's milk and 5–8 percent of human milk. All fresh (non-fermented) dairy products are a source of lactose.

Like the disaccharide sucrose, maltose and lactose add some sweetness to foods.

Sweeteners

One of the purposes, and the appeal, of sugar in foods is sweetness. Food manufacturers add sugar to many of their processed foods to make these foods more palatable. Manufacturers often use a variety of terms that all mean the same thing: some sugar has been added to this product. The following terms are all used for added sugar:

➤ Sugar, confectioner's sugar, brown sugar, invert sugar, or date sugar

➤ Sucrose

➤ Dextrose (the same thing as glucose)

➤ Fructose, fruit sugar, or levulose (they all mean the same thing)

➤ Lactose

➤ Corn syrup (contains mainly oligosaccharides and maltose)

➤ High-fructose corn syrup (HFCS) (a mixture of about 55 percent fructose, 42 percent glucose, and 3 percent other sweeteners)

➤ Honey, molasses, maple syrup, or caramel

➤ Sorbitol or xylitol (known as sugar alcohols)

➤ Polydextrose or maltodextrins (a fancy way of saying "lots of glucose")

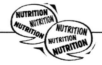

Nutrition Vocabulary

Invert sugar is sucrose that has been treated to break apart into its components, glucose and fructose. By breaking apart the chemical into its constituents, invert sugar tastes slightly sweeter than sucrose.

The above chemicals give you some calories of energy when you eat them. In the past several decades, food manufacturers have invented new chemicals to sweeten food but the body cannot get any energy out of them at all. They have little or no calories. These are called alternative sweeteners:

➤ Saccharin (sold as Sweet'N Low)

➤ Aspartame (sold as Equal and NutraSweet)

➤ Sucralose (sold as Splenda)

➤ Neotame

➤ Acesulfame-K (sold as Sunett or Sweet One)

➤ Tagatose (sold as Naturlose and Shugr)

➤ Stevia plant extracts (sold as SweetLeaf and Truvia)

➤ Cyclamates (banned in the United States for potential safety reasons, but sold elsewhere)

Because sucrose, lactose, and the other calorie-containing sweeteners can be used in body metabolism, nutritionists call them nutritive sweeteners. The alternative sweeteners listed above are non-nutritive sweeteners.

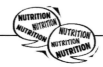

Nutrition Vocabulary

Sugar alcohols have chemical structures similar to sugars, but they all contain an alcohol portion made of an oxygen connected to hydrogen. Chemists write this *-OH*. The body does not use sugar alcohols as readily as it uses regular sugars, so these chemicals deliver few or no calories. Common sugar alcohols in foods are: sorbitol, xylitol, mannitol, lactitol, maltitol, isomalt, glycerol, and hydrogenated starch hydrolysate (HSH).

The Sweetness Index

Since the whole purpose of adding sugar or a sweetener is to make food taste sweeter than natural, manufacturers have devised a ranking system for all the sweet things they put in drinks, waffles, spaghetti sauce, and so on. The sweetness index is based on the sweetness of sucrose, which is given a value of 1.0. Values higher than 1 are sweeter than sucrose; values lower than 1 are less sweet than sucrose:

➤ Lactose: 0.2

➤ Maltose: 0.4

➤ Glucose: 0.7

➤ Sugar alcohols: 0.6–0.9

➤ Tagalose: 0.9–1.5

➤ Invert sugar: 1.3

➤ Fructose: 1.7

➤ Aspartame: 180

➤ Saccharin: 300

➤ Sucralose: 600

➤ Neotame: 7,000–13,000

Nutrition Morsels

High-fructose corn syrup (HCFS) is one of the most common sweeteners added to processed foods. HFCS contains more than 50 percent fructose, which is readily available to be absorbed by the digestive tract. By contrast, the fructose in table sugar must be liberated by enzymes from the sucrose molecule, a step that slows down the influx of sugar into the bloodstream.

Once fructose in the bloodstream gets taken up by cells, it may be used for energy—just like glucose—or put into storage. Unlike glucose, which gets stored in glycogen, fructose might be stored only as fat. Students at Princeton University recently showed that rats fed water sweetened with HFCS gained significantly more weight and fat than rats fed the same number of calories in water sweetened with table sugar.

What Happens When You Get Too Much Sugar

A diet imbalanced by the intake of too much sugar leads to trouble. Some of the well-known hazards to high sugar intake are:

➤ Dental caries: Sugars and starches increase the likelihood of developing tooth decay due to the fermentation of the sugars into acid by bacteria in the mouth.

➤ Diabetes: A disease that has more than one form, all characterized by the inability to properly control glucose levels in the bloodstream.

➤ Hypoglycemia: The body's reaction to a sharp increase in sugar intake by removing as much glucose from the blood as possible. This causes an overproduction of the hormone insulin, which reduces blood sugar too much, leading to irritability, headache, and nervousness.

High-sugar diets have been linked to hyperactivity in children. Some literature specifically states that these diets may lead to attention deficit hyperactivity disorder (ADHD). There has never been a definitive connection between high-sugar diets and the medical condition of hyperactivity. High-sugar diets, nevertheless, decrease any diet's quality by:

➤ Reducing the room for other nutrients; that is, reducing the nutrient density of your diet

➤ Increasing the energy density of your diet, causing you to take in more calories relative to nutrients

Glycemic Index

Nutritionists rate the relative health hazards of sugar foods by assigning each food a value on a scale called the glycemic index. On the glycemic index, foods with a low score have small effects on blood glucose fluctuations. Foods with higher scores on the index cause greater fluctuations in blood glucose and insulin levels soon after each meal. The index ranges from 0 to 100, where glucose has a score of 100. For better health, you should strive for foods with lower glycemic index scores.

The Harvard Medical School publishes a glycemic index list at www.health.harvard.edu/ newsweek/Glycemic_index_and_glycemic_load_for_100_foods.htm.

A glycemic index score is just a number. What does it mean to you in practical nutrition? To relate the glycemic index to your personal energy needs, consider the following scale:

➤ High scores of 70–100 relate to foods that give your body a quick and sudden influx of sugar. You might crave these foods after very strenuous exercise because your blood sugar levels have been lowered. Examples are white bread, pastries, chocolate cake, mashed potatoes, baked potato, instant white rice, corn flakes, dates, and watermelon.

➤ Medium scores of 56–69 relate to foods that are good sources of sugar but release the sugar slowly from the digestive tract into the bloodstream. These are useful foods for supplying energy if kept in balance with protein and fat intake. Examples are rye bread, oatmeal, chocolate (dark) bar, beets, most granola energy bars, pineapple, and raisins.

➤ Low scores of less than 55 relate to foods that give you little sugar but still can be used for energy. Low glycemic index foods are good for losing weight, controlling diabetes, lowering blood cholesterol, and reducing risk of heart disease. Examples are bran cereal, barley, converted rice, whole wheat pasta, beans (cooked dry beans, not canned), popcorn (no butter), peanuts, grapefruit, and low-fat yogurt and milk.

Glycemic Load

You may also notice the term *glycemic load* when looking up the glycemic index of particular foods. Glycemic load helps you get an idea of the sugar intake you get from specific foods based on the food's serving size.

Glycemic load equals the amount of carbohydrate in a serving multiplied by the glycemic index of the food's carbohydrate, then divided by 100. If for example, a serving of spaghetti contains 40 grams of carbohydrate and a glycemic index of 41, the glycemic load is:

$$(40 \times 41) \div 100 = 16.4$$

Nutrition Morsels

A person's ideal blood sugar level (also called plasma glucose) is between 70 and 99 milligrams (mg) per 10 milliliters (ml) of blood. (In the metric system, 10 ml is the same as 1 deciliter, or dl, and doctors often report blood sugars levels as so many mg per dl.) After a meal, blood sugar rises for a few hours and then returns to its normal range as the body's cells absorb glucose.

Blood glucose levels below 70 mg/dl indicate hypoglycemia. When glucose levels rise above about 150 mg/dl, the condition is called hyperglycemia. A blood glucose level of 126 mg/dl is the threshold for diabetes. You may not necessarily have diabetes, but your doctor will view this blood sugar level as a warning sign that you may be predisposed to developing diabetes in the future.

The following gives examples of where some foods fall on the glycemic load scale.

➤ Peanuts (1 serving): 14

➤ Apple (1): 38

➤ Banana (1): 51

➤ Cola (1 can): 58

➤ Sweet potato (1): 61

➤ Rice cake (1): 78

➤ Corn flakes (1 serving): 81

➤ Baguette (1): 95

Glycemic index and load provide ways of putting a number on slow sugar versus fast sugar.

CHAPTER 10

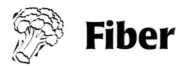 **Fiber**

In This Chapter

➤ Types of fiber and how they relate to carbohydrates
➤ How fiber is digested
➤ How fiber benefits health and overall nutrition

In this chapter you learn the benefits of fiber as well as what fiber is, how it relates to carbohydrates, and how it plays a role in good nutrition.

We all hear lately that we must get more fiber in our diet. How much fiber are we getting now? Why isn't it enough, and can we get too much of it? This chapter will answer these questions as well as describe the types of fiber you ingest and how the body digests fiber.

Is Fiber a Carbohydrate?

Many nutrition books discuss fiber along with carbohydrates for the simple reason that fibers are made of many sugars linked together. This makes fiber seem like it might behave like a carbohydrate in nutrition, but, in fact, fiber plays a very different role from carbohydrates in human nutrition.

Fiber is the term for a variety of substances in plants that cannot be degraded by the human digestive tract. (Fiber found naturally in plant foods is often called dietary fiber.)

Fiber is strong. It gives plants the ability to stand upright and even withstand much of the damage of insects and animals that try to munch on plant stalks and leaves. Fiber's strength comes from the manner in which its sugars and sugar-like substances bond together chemically. Not only does this chemical bond strengthen fiber, it makes it difficult to digest by the enzymes that easily break apart polysaccharides, oligosaccharides, and shorter sugar chains. So although at first glance fiber looks like a carbohydrate such as starch, it actually differs in its chemical properties. These chemical properties in turn make fiber behave much differently from starches once it gets ingested by an animal.

So, don't be surprised if you find one nutrition book that discusses fiber right along with carbohydrates, and another book that separates carbohydrates and fiber into two distinct nutrient groups.

Types of Dietary Fiber

Nutritionists divide dietary fiber into two main groups based on how well they dissolve in water:

> Insoluble fibers: Cellulose, hemicelluloses, and lignin

> Soluble fibers: Pectins, gums, and mucilages

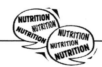

Nutrition Vocabulary

Cellulose is composed of long, straight chains of glucoses linked together. Chemists call their chemical bond a beta linkage, which is very difficult to break down in nature and gives cellulose its strength.

Hemicellulose refers to a variety of fibers made from a mixture of six-carbon and five-carbon sugars. Hemicelluloses all contain glucose, but the main sugar in all of these fibers is the five-carbon sugar xylose. Another difference from cellulose is hemicellulose's extensive branching into many side chains.

Both cellulose and the hemicelluloses make up the rigid outer wall of plant cells.

All fibers, especially insoluble fibers, add bulk to the material that passes through the digestive tract. As you will soon see, this bulk helps with digestion and the health of the digestive tract. Insoluble fiber sources are stalk vegetables, such as broccoli and celery, legumes, root vegetables (tubers), and whole grains. Soluble fibers are found in fruits and berries in both the skin and fleshy portions.

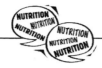

Nutrition Vocabulary

Legumes are plants that develop a fruit or reproductive structure in a pod. Common legumes in your diet are peas, chickpeas, beans, soybeans and edamame, lentils, and peanuts. Other legumes important in livestock diets are alfalfa and clover.

Our digestive tract can break down the various fibers differently. Lignin is virtually indestructible by us and by most other digestive tracts. By comparison, we do a fairly good job breaking apart pectins in our intestines.

Nutritionists put fibers into different classifications based on how they are broken down in the human digestive tract:

➤ Functional fiber: Largely undigestible but able to give the body health benefits by contributing to bulk in the digestive tract.

➤ Viscous fiber: Fiber that can be broken down at least partially in the digestive tract. Most of this breakdown is done by intestinal bacteria rather than enzymes secreted by the body.

➤ Total fiber: The sum of functional and viscous fiber.

Some nutritionists who prefer to include fibers with carbohydrates use another classification scheme:

➤ Fermentable: Fibers that bacteria in your digestive tract can digest partially or entirely, such as polysaccharides, gums, mucilages, and pectins. (Some hemicelluloses also belong to this group.)

➤ Non-fermentable: Fibers that bacteria have a hard time degrading, such as lignin, cellulose, and many hemicelluloses.

Digesting Dietary Fiber

Humans and other animals with similar digestive systems do not digest fibers particularly well. Most fiber goes from the mouth to the anus undigested.

Humans have a monogastric digestive system, which is not suited to digesting large amounts of fiber. Even animals that live entirely on plant foods (herbivores) do not digest fibers directly. These animals rely on their huge populations of bacteria in the digestive tract to do the work of breaking down plant fibers to glucose and other end products. Only lignin moves through herbivore digestive tracts largely untouched as it does through non-herbivore, or monogastric, digestive tracts.

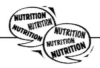

Nutrition Vocabulary

Monogastric digestive tracts consist of a single acid-secreting stomach. Foods that have been partially digested in the mouth and by stomach acids move to the small intestine and then to the large intestine for further breakdown and absorption of nutrients. Animals with monogastric digestive tracts are carnivores and omnivores. This group includes humans, swine, dogs, cats, and rats and mice.

When digestive tract bacteria break down some of the fiber you ingest, they release glucose. These bacteria use up most of this glucose for their own growth, but any leftover glucose gets absorbed by the digestive tract and goes into the bloodstream. In this way, the glucose you get from fiber is used by your body exactly the same way as glucose from a potato or an ear of corn or a candy bar.

Nutrition Morsels

Ruminant animals are those that have a multi-compartment stomach (called the rumen) that acts as a large fermentation vat for breaking down plant fiber. Ruminant animals, such as cattle, sheep, goats, deer, moose, giraffes, and elephants, grind plant materials in their mouths, which are equipped with large, flat teeth. It takes a lot of grinding to chew plants high in lignin. That's why ruminants spend a lot of their time—about a third of their day—chewing the cud. By chewing the plant, the animal breaks up lignin to help release more digestible fibers and carbohydrates that intact lignin normally protects.

The plant matter then goes to the rumen, where a diverse population of bacteria and protozoa ferment the fibers, similar to how fibers are fermented in winemaking and brewing. These fermentations produce acids from the fibers' sugars. Ruminant animals then absorb the acids and use them for energy and for making any glucose needed by the animal.

The Role of Dietary Fiber in Nutrition

First of all we must answer the question, "is fiber a nutrient?" If humans cannot digest fiber, then how could it be considered a nutrient that helps us grow, move, reproduce, and maintain basic body functions?

Because fiber has been shown to give your digestion some benefits, nutritionists give it a sort of honorary status as a nutrient. You get almost no energy or essential chemicals directly from fiber, but fiber helps with overall digestion and nutrition. Fiber does this by adding bulk to the diet. In other words, fiber takes up space in foods and in the digestive tract. Bulk is good for three reasons:

> ➤ It helps lower the energy density of foods. By doing this, you take in fewer calories relative to other nutrients.

> ➤ It fills you up. While bulk lowers energy density it also gives you a feeling of fullness because fiber absorbs water. This helps reduce your inclination to overeat.

> ➤ Bulk activates the intestinal waves of peristalsis. Peristalsis prevents your digestive tract from clogging up. As a result, a steady flow of undigested food and fiber helps make room for the next meal and its bounty of nutrients.

Since the discovery that fiber enhances overall nutrition, doctors and nutritionists have studied other ways that fiber might indirectly benefit health.

Some of the benefits believed to come from dietary fiber are:

> ➤ Helping with weight control by reducing calorie intake

> ➤ Stabilizing blood sugar levels and thus helping to control or prevent diabetes

> ➤ Lowering the risk of heart disease, which may be connected to fiber's effect on blood levels of fats and cholesterol

Nutrition Vocabulary

Whole grains are grains such as wheat, rye, corn, oats, barley, and rice that contain the entire seed produced by a plant. A whole seed consists of three parts:

1. The bran or tough outer coat

2. The germ, the softer portion of the seed from which a new plant arises

3. The endosperm, the starchy food supply for a young plant.

Whole grains can be cracked, crushed, or flaked. But to give you the same benefit as the original grain, they should contain bran, germ, and endosperm in the same proportions as unadulterated grain.

> ➤ Reducing the risk of numerous bowel diseases, such as diverticulitis, hemorrhoids, polyps, colon cancer, and irritable bowel syndrome

> ➤ Correcting constipation, particularly in the elderly

How Much Fiber Do I Need?

Researchers have set our fiber requirements based on the ability to reduce heart disease. For a person eating about 2,000 kcal per day, daily fiber requirements are:

> ➤ Up to age 50: 25 grams for women; 38 grams for men

> ➤ After age 50: 21 grams for women; 30 grams for men

Most Americans do get enough fiber in their diet. Nutritionists estimate that women get about 13 grams of fiber a day, and men get about 17 grams per day.

The best sources of dietary fiber are fresh vegetables, fruits, whole grains, whole grain cereals and snack bars, and granola. Other ways to increase fiber intake is to substitute whole wheat pasta for regular pasta, brown rice for white rice, fresh fruit for fruit juice, legumes for meat about three times a week, and snack on raw vegetables instead of chips and candy.

Too Much Fiber

Nutrition is chock full of examples of too much of a good thing. This is true for fiber, too. A diet imbalanced by too much fiber can cause the following problems:

> ➤ Constipation, unless you drink a lot more fluids with high-fiber meals.

> ➤ Decreased nutrient uptake by the decreased efficiency of intestinal movement and absorption. Fiber binds to some nutrients, such as minerals, and reduces their absorption from the intestines.

> ➤ Inadequate energy intake, especially in children.

> ➤ Stomach and intestinal irritation—fiber is scratchy!

CHAPTER 11

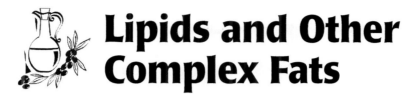 **Lipids and Other Complex Fats**

In this chapter you will learn what a lipid is, the difference between lipids and fat, and the purpose of lipids in the body. As with other chapters in this book devoted to a single group of nutrients, I describe how people digest lipids, how we store them in the body, and how we use them for energy and other jobs.

Understanding the lipids in your food and the ones that wind up in your blood is important. Lipid levels are associated with cardiovascular diseases, which are diseases that affect the heart and/or the arteries. Coronary heart disease involves specifically the coronary arteries, which are the main vessels that supply blood to the heart. Dietary lipids have been linked to the incidence of cardiovascular disease and coronary heart disease in North America.

What Makes It a Lipid?

A lipid is a chemical made of mostly carbon and hydrogen, a little oxygen, and sometimes a few other atoms. The high proportion of carbon and hydrogen makes all lipids insoluble in water.

The major groups of lipids found in nature and also in your diet are:

➤ Fats: Discussed in more detail in the next chapter, fats include fatty acids and triglycerides. They are common in many foods, and fats in your body become the main long-term storage form of energy. Fats are solid at room temperature; think butter and lard!

➤ Oils: Similar in composition to fats, oils are liquid at room temperature.

➤ Cholesterol: This lipid has a bad reputation because of the relationship of blood cholesterol levels to coronary heart disease. Cholesterol is nevertheless essential to your body.

➤ Compound lipids: These lipids are always attached to another chemical, such as a sugar (glycolipids) or a phosphate (phospholipids). Complex lipids are important because they enable cells to communicate with each other and ensure proper nerve function. They are also a component of brain and nerve tissue, and membranes.

➤ Waxes: Probably not a big part of your diet. Waxes are solid at room temperature. They are part of beeswax and the coating on apple skins.

Nature also produces two additional types of lipids that play a very minor role in nutrition. These are prostaglandins and terpenes, described later in this chapter.

Glycerol and Lipids

Nutritionists sometimes categorize lipids based on whether the lipid is built on a three-carbon chemical called glycerol. By this classification scheme, your diet contains glycerol-based lipids and non-glycerol-based lipids:

➤ Glycerol-based lipids: Simple lipids (called fats) and complex lipids (called compound lipids). Compound lipids are glycolipids and phospholipids.

➤ Non-glycerol-based lipids: Sterols and waxes.

Cholesterol

Cholesterol is a waxy substance found in all cells of your body. It comes only from foods of animal origin; fruits, vegetables, and grains do not have cholesterol in them. You get cholesterol from meat, eggs, dairy products, and seafood and shellfish. The body also makes its own cholesterol. Therefore, your blood cholesterol levels come from a combination of dietary cholesterol and the cholesterol made naturally by your body. (The brain is unique in the body because it cannot use dietary cholesterol and depends entirely on the cholesterol it produces.)

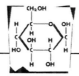

The Chemistry of Nutrition

Sterols are organic chemicals that all belong to the same classification because of their chemical structure. All sterols are built of carbon atoms arranged in rings. Chemists call any compound that has this multi-ring structure a steroid. In addition to the steroid rings, all sterols have a hydroxyl group, which is simply an oxygen atom attached to a hydrogen. Chemists abbreviate it as -OH.

Cholesterol is a typical example of a sterol that is important in your body. Other sterols that play a role in metabolism are hormones, bile acids, and vitamin D. The hormones based on sterol are called steroid hormones. These include testosterone, estrogen, progesterone, and glucocorticoids.

What Lipids Do in the Body

Lipids are a diverse group of chemicals. Their inability to dissolve in water is one of the few traits they all have in common. Therefore, when considering what lipids do in the body, you must focus on a particular lipid. Cholesterol, for instance, has several vital roles in health. The main jobs of lipids other than cholesterol are:

➤ Fats: Energy and carbon storage. Adipose tissue protects internal body organs, such as the spleen, kidneys, liver, and heart. This tissue also insulates the body against too much heat loss. At very cold temperatures, you burn fat to generate additional heat.

➤ Fatty acids: Energy storage, immune system function, production of hormone-like substances in the body, constituent of cell membranes, and aid in the digestion and uptake of other fats.

➤ Glycolipids: Components of cell membranes, these chemicals stick out from the cell thereby making the cell recognizable to other cells or to the immune system. Your blood type (A, B, AB, or O) is determined by the array of glycolipids attached to your red blood cells.

➤ Phospholipids: Provide a chemical structure for making lecithin, which is used in emulsifying fats inside the digestive tract, and cephalin, which is instrumental in helping nerve cells work.

Nutrition Morsels

Cholesterol has more jobs in the body than most other lipids. Yet we think of cholesterol as a bad thing. That's why you might hear the terms *good cholesterol* and *bad cholesterol* to distinguish between the cholesterol that works for you and the cholesterol that works against you.

Good cholesterol is the cholesterol traveling through the bloodstream in high density lipoproteins (HDL). HDL benefits you by taking excess cholesterol out of body tissues and transporting it to the liver, which will help get it out of the body. Bad cholesterol travels through the bloodstream in low density lipoproteins (LDL). LDLs build up on the inner walls of arteries and can eventually clog them. This leads to heart attack and other possibly fatal health events.

Blood levels of individual LDLs and HDLs are important to your health, but even more important are the ratios of these lipoproteins to each other. You should try to reach the following levels for good and bad cholesterol: 60 mg/dl or more of HDL; less than 100 mg/dl of LDL; and a HDL:LDL ratio of above 0.3 or 0.4. (If the blood test reverses the ratio to LDL:HDL, then the desirable range is 1 to 2 and no higher than 3.)

The diverse roles of cholesterol (good cholesterol) in the body are:

> ➤ Strengthens membranes

> ➤ Helps to control which substances enter and exit cells

> ➤ Insulates nerve cells

> ➤ Serves as a precursor for several hormones and vitamin D

> ➤ Aids in fat digestion by being a precursor to bile salts

> ➤ Helps the body use vitamins A, D, E, and K

Like most nutrients, you can get too much cholesterol in your diet. As a result, cholesterol builds up in the body and goes from being a necessary nutrient to a potential killer. To understand the hazards of cholesterol, you must know a little about substances in your blood called lipoproteins.

Cholesterol and Lipoproteins

It is difficult to discuss cholesterol's activities in the body without also thinking about another lipid-like substance called lipoprotein. A lipoprotein is a chemical made of both protein and lipids.

Four different types of lipoproteins serve the body by helping transport fats throughout the bloodstream. Because fats cannot dissolve in blood, lipoproteins are essential for delivering fats to tissues. Lipoproteins also play an important role in the cholesterol levels of your blood. Here's how the four lipoproteins work:

➤ Chylomicrons: The least dense droplets, they are made mainly of triglycerides. The body uses them to carry dietary fat from the intestines to cells.

➤ Very low density lipoproteins (VLDL): Also made of triglycerides, VLDL carry lipids from the liver to other tissues.

➤ Low density lipoproteins (LDL): Composed mainly of cholesterol, these lipoproteins carry dietary cholesterol to all cells.

➤ High density lipoproteins (HDL): The densest droplets, HDLs remove cholesterol from tissues and help clear cholesterol from the body.

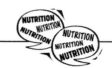

Nutrition Vocabulary

Lipoproteins are constituents of blood. They are ball-like droplets containing a lipid core enclosed in a shell made of protein, cholesterol, and phospholipids.

From the jobs of lipoproteins listed above, you can probably figure out that LDLs are also called bad cholesterol and HDLs are thought of as good cholesterol. VLDLs may be included with bad cholesterol because they have a tendency to absorb cholesterol and clog arteries in the same way LDLs damage your blood vessels.

Health Hazards of Bad Cholesterol

Bad cholesterol circulating at high levels in your bloodstream leads to the following problems:

➤ High risk of coronary heart disease and/or heart attack

➤ Atherosclerosis, a narrowing of the arteries

➤ Angina, an inadequate oxygen supply to heart muscle, causing pain

➤ Loss of elasticity of the blood vessels

➤ Stroke

Nutrition Morsels

Blood cholesterol is measured in milligrams per deciliter (mg/dl) the same as blood glucose levels. For good health, you should strive to keep cholesterol levels below 200 mg/dl and triglyceride levels below 150 mg/dl. Dangerously high blood cholesterol levels start at 240 mg/dl. Borderline levels are between 200 and 239 mg/dl.

You cannot control the cholesterol made by your body, but you can control your intake of dietary cholesterol.

The best way to lower bad cholesterol blood levels and increase the proportion of good cholesterol is to decrease foods of animal origin in your diet while increasing the proportions of beans, whole grains, raw vegetables, and fruits.

How We Digest Lipids

Lipids are harder to digest than most other nutrients because they do not dissolve in the watery contents of your intestines. Being insoluble also makes them more difficult to absorb through the intestinal lining. In fact, your body hardly absorbs any waxes and few of the sterols. It does a much better job digesting and absorbing simple lipids.

Lipid digestion starts in the stomach, where the enzyme lipase begins breaking down many lipids. (The saliva also has a little bit of lipase, but it's not enough to matter; no significant lipid breakdown occurs in the mouth.)

Digestion continues in the small intestine, where lipase from the pancreas converts the lipids into tiny globules. The formation of these globules is helped by bile salts from the gall bladder. Bile salts attach to the outside of the globules, and by doing so they help keep the lipids suspended in the intestinal contents. This act of suspending an insoluble substance in water is called emulsification.

Both bile salts and lecithin break down large fat globules into smaller ones. This increases the globules' surface area, which gives the lipase a better shot at digesting more of the lipid. As the digestion continues, the globules become smaller and smaller until they are tiny— almost microscopic—droplets called micelles.

As lipase chews on the suspended micelles, triglycerides get broken down into glycerol and fatty acids. The intestinal lining then absorbs these.

All the absorbed lipids go to the liver. Small lipids go directly to the liver via the portal vein; larger lipids are carried in the body's lymph, but they too eventually find the liver.

How We Store Lipids

The liver has two choices regarding what to do with the glycerol, fatty acids, and other lipids that come its way: package the lipids for storage or use them immediately for energy.

If the liver decides to store fat, it first reassembles the triglycerides. Even though you just digested the triglycerides in the diet to small pieces to be absorbed, the liver reconnects fatty acids to the glycerol to reform triglycerides. Chylomicrons then transport the triglycerides from the liver to adipose tissue.

Adipose tissue is more than 80 percent triglycerides and about 15 percent water. It also holds a small amount of protein, potassium, and sodium.

Lipids in the Body

Lipids move into and out of your cells and blood depending on your level of activity and energy needs. When you have a blood test done to determine your blood lipid levels, no single lipid indicates your overall health. Your doctor will look at your cholesterol, triglycerides, and lipoproteins, as well as the ratios of these components. In addition, blood glucose levels relate to fat stores because both glucose and fat serve as your main energy sources. Of course, other blood components, such as liver enzymes and nitrogen-containing wastes will give an indication of liver and kidney function, respectively.

Blood Lipid Profiles

Let's look at the blood components that indicate whether your lipid metabolism is in or out of balance. In blood testing, this group of values is called a lipid profile. Your doctor evaluates each component of the lipid profile and their relationship to each other to decide if you are at risk for developing atherosclerosis and/or coronary heart disease.

The lipid profile has five main components:

1. Total cholesterol: This value is directly linked to your risk of developing heart or blood vessel disease. People over the age of twenty-one should try to keep cholesterol levels between 100 and 199 mg/dl. People twenty years of age or younger should have total cholesterol levels in the range of 75–169 mg/dl.

2. Triglycerides: These are also indicators of potentially impending heart or coronary disease. High triglycerides also appear in people who are very overweight, obese, or diabetic. Try to keep your triglyceride levels below 150 mg/dl. Levels less than 130 mg/dl are desirable and levels above 200 mg/dl are dangerous.

3. HDL cholesterol: This is the good cholesterol in which high levels in your blood help reduce your risk of heart or coronary disease. Keep your HDL levels above 40 mg/dl.

4. LDL cholesterol: For good health, you want to lower your blood levels of LDL. High blood levels of LDL are known to link directly to heart and coronary disease, diseases of other blood vessels, heart attacks, and death. Target blood LDL levels of less than 130 mg/dl if

you are a healthy individual. If your doctor has already told you that you have a high risk of heart or coronary disease, you should keep your LDL levels below 100 mg/dl. People who have already experienced any heart-related disease should keep their LDL levels below 70 mg/dl for continued good health.

5. Total cholesterol, HDL ratio: This is another way of assessing your risks of heart and coronary disease. Many doctors believe the ratio is a better indicator of cardiovascular disease than total cholesterol levels. For men, a ratio of 5.0 indicates average risk and for women average risk is 4.5. Your risk of cardiovascular disease decreases as the ratio decreases. Any ratio in double digits indicates a high risk for trouble.

Nutrition Morsels

How do you control the levels of tiny fat droplets circulating through your blood without obsessing about blood tests? In fact, how do you sleep after reading this chapter? Fortunately, researchers have done a lot of studies on the best ways of raising your good cholesterol while simultaneously lowering bad cholesterol.

To increase the good HDLs in your blood, quit smoking, lose weight, and increase your amount of exercise. To decrease the bad LDLs, decrease saturated fat intake (see next chapter), increase dietary fiber, increase your amount of strenuous (aerobic) exercise, and maintain good body composition by reducing percent fat and building more muscle.

Other Blood Components Related to Lipids

If your lipid profile contains warning signs that you have a higher than normal risk of disease, your doctor may test for additional factors in your blood. These factors give a fuller picture of your body's lipid metabolism:

➤ Lipoprotein(a): This lipoprotein may be related to higher risks for heart attack and stroke. The target level for most adults is below 30 mg/dl.

➤ Apolipoprotein A-1: Apolipoproteins are proteins imbedded in the outer coating of your blood's lipoproteins. A-1 is a major component of HDL. Therefore, doctors recommend you keep your ApoA1 levels above 123 mg/dl.

➤ Apolipoprotein B: Apo B is an indicator of your LDL levels because it is a component of this type of lipoprotein. Most healthy people should try to keep their apo B levels below 100 mg/dl, but people with a high risk of heart disease or diabetes should strive for levels below 80 mg/dl.

➤ LDL-associated phospholipase A_2: This is an enzyme (abbreviated LDL-associated PLA2) that might indicate damage to the body's blood vessels. This enzyme is measured in very small amounts in the blood; values are usually shown as nanograms (ng) per milliliter (ml) of blood. The desirable range is 200–235 ng/ml.

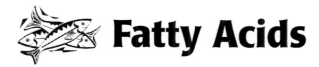

CHAPTER 12

Fatty Acids

> ## In This Chapter
>
> ➤ Types of fats and fatty acids
>
> ➤ Essential fatty acids and what they do for you
>
> ➤ How to choose the best fats and avoid bad fats

In this chapter you are introduced to fatty acids, specialized lipids that give you energy and also store energy. When too many fatty acids accumulate to store energy, however, your waistline expands!

By understanding how fatty acids move into and out of your body fat, you might feel more in charge of them. Let's make those fatty acids work for you instead of letting them sit around in adipose tissue!

Meet the Fats

Sometimes we use the terms *fat* and *lipid* interchangeably. In reality, a fat is a type of lipid. To a chemist, a fat is a glyceride, which is a glycerol molecule that holds one, two, or three fatty acids.

Picture a hair comb with only three teeth. Glycerol makes up the comb's backbone. The three teeth extending from the glycerol are fatty acids. Thus, chemists use the word *triglyceride* to describe a glycerol that is holding three fatty acids. (The correct chemical term is *triacylglycerol*.) The fatty acids can all be the same type or different.

Now break off one of the teeth. Missing one of the fatty acids, you have just made a diglyceride. Diglycerides are a glycerol holding two fatty acids. Break off another fatty acid and you now have a monoglyceride.

Fat cells that make up adipose tissue (adipocytes) contain mostly triglycerides and lesser amounts of di- and monoglycerides. Triglycerides fill up adipocytes until these cells swell to round balloon-like globs. So many triglycerides can fill the middle of a cell that the other parts of the cell get squished into a narrow region, kind of like an overstuffed jelly doughnut.

Glycerol is the same chemical that gives all fats their framework. The fats in your diet and those that are deposited in places around your body differ by the types of fatty acids attached to the glycerol molecule.

Nutrition Morsels

When you increase your exercise, your body adjusts to a need for generating extra energy. For a while, your body doesn't think you're serious about this exercise thing. It takes some glucose from glycogen and gives the glucose to cells that need more energy. But if you keep exercising, your body gets the message and begins withdrawing from your energy bank account: the fat in adipose tissue. This is why a sustained exercise regimen improves health better than sporadic bursts of short-duration exercise.

Fatty Acids

Fatty acids are chains of carbon linked to each other in a row, most carrying a hydrogen atom. In this way, fatty acids seem very similar to carbohydrates such as polysaccharides. But fats differ from carbohydrates by having very little oxygen. From the shortest fatty acids to the longest, a fatty acid contains only two oxygen atoms at its tail. The long carbon-hydrogen chain cannot dissolve in water. Only the oxygen-containing end has a small attraction to water, but usually not enough to dissolve the rest of the long fatty acid.

Fatty acids usually contain an even number of carbons. They range from two to more than thirty carbons in a single fatty acid chain. (Nature rarely has fatty acids of longer than thirty-six carbons.)

Some of the most common fatty acids in the diet come from specific foods. For instance, acetic acid (two carbons) is the main constituent of vinegar; butyric acid (four) is common in milk fats such as butter; and caproic acid (six) shows up in goat's milk.

Fatty acids with carbon chain lengths greater than eighteen (written C_{18} or C18) are uncommon in nature. The most common fatty acid lengths in your diet are from C14 to C18 in even numbers of carbon atoms. These fatty acids are myristic acid (C14), palmitic acid (C16), and stearic acid (C18).

Fatty acids are responsible for the rancid smell of fatty foods when they become spoiled. Even unspoiled, fatty acids of about C8 and shorter can dissipate into the air. We perceive these chemicals as bad smells. Thus, fatty acids give goat's and sheep's milk their strong odors and do the same for many of the world's smelliest cheeses.

Fatty Acids for Energy

The body breaks down fats to carbon dioxide and water. In this process, called beta-oxidation (β-oxidation), fats get burned for energy production the same way the body uses glucose. When the body needs to make new fatty acids, it takes some of the carbons from glucose.

Even when the body doesn't need to store any more fat, it still does if your diet is high in carbohydrates! Excess glucose entering the liver gets converted into fatty acids. The fatty acids are then assembled onto glycerol molecules to make triglycerides, and then shipped off to adipose tissue.

The hormone insulin, which helps control blood sugar levels, also activates fat deposition. This is why high-carbohydrate diets lead to weight gain.

Saturated, Monounsaturated, and Polyunsaturated Fats

Food chemists—scientists who study the chemical makeup of food—divide fatty acids into two main groups: saturated and unsaturated. The carbons of saturated fatty acids are completely filled up with hydrogen atoms. Saturated fatty acids are common in the meat and milk products of ruminant animals (beef, lamb, and cow's milk, goat's milk, and sheep's milk).

Unsaturated fatty acids have one or more carbons that are not filled up with hydrogens. Instead, two adjacent carbons form what chemists call a double carbon bond. If you were to imagine a regular carbon-to-carbon bond as -C-C-, you could picture a carbon double bond as -C=C-.

Saturated Fats

Saturated fats are triglycerides containing saturated fatty acids attached to their glycerol backbone. Saturated fats are the main type of fat you get from red meats, such as beef, lamb, bison, and venison. These meat-producing animals are ruminant animals. Due to the type of chemical reactions carried out by bacteria in their big fermentation organ, the rumen, these animals turn all dietary fats into saturated fat.

The predominant saturated fatty acids of the diet are shown below. Chemists describe these fatty acids in shorthand to signify the number of carbons in the chain. For example, palmitic acid is written C16:0, which means that this specific fatty acid has sixteen carbons and zero double bonds.

➤ Acetic acid (C2:0): Ruminant animals use this fat for energy so none will be found in meat, but you get acetic acid in your diet from vinegar.

➤ Butyric acid (C4:0): Common in milk fats such as butter.

➤ Caproic acid (C6:0): A main fatty acid of goat's milk, butter, and coconut oil.

➤ Caprylic acid (C8:0): Common in both animal and vegetable fats, especially coconut oil.

➤ Capric acid (C10:0): Found in coconut oil, butter, and goat's milk.

➤ Lauric acid (C12:0): The predominant fatty acid in coconut oil as well as palm and cinnamon oils.

➤ Myristic acid (C14:0): Found in coconut oil, butter, tallow, safflower oil, and eggs.

➤ Palmitic acid (C16:0): Most common fatty acid of plants and animals. In butter, tallow, safflower oil, soy, corn oil, coconut oil, lard, and eggs.

➤ Stearic acid (C18:0): Widespread in fats and oils similar to palmitic acid and also found in cocoa.

➤ Arachidic acid (C20:0): Found in some seeds and in low levels in milk fat.

➤ Behenic acid (C22:0): Found in ben oil and almost nowhere else.

➤ Lignoceric acid (C24:0): Found in legume seed oils and few other places.

Myristic, palmitic, and stearic acids are the most common saturated fatty acids in our diets.

Unsaturated Fats

If a fatty acid contains only one double carbon-to-carbon bond somewhere along its carbon chain, the fatty acid is called monounsaturated. When the unsaturated fatty acid contains more than one double bond, it is called polyunsaturated. The shorthand for these fatty acids follows the same formula as used for saturated fatty acids. For example, the formula C18:3 describes a fatty acid that is made of eighteen carbons and the carbon chain contains three double bonds.

Unsaturated fats are found in vegetable oils and the fats of meat-producing animals that are not ruminant animals. Thus, chicken, fish, and shellfish have more unsaturated fats than red meat.

Some common dietary unsaturated fatty acids are:

➤ Myristoleic acid (C14:1)

➤ Palmitoleic (C16:1)

➤ Oleic acid (C18:1)

➤ Linoleic (C18:2)

➤ Linolenic acid (C18:3)

➤ Arachidonic acid (C20:4)

Myristoleic, palmitoleic, and oleic acids are monounsaturated acids. Linoleic, linolenic, and arachidonic acids are polyunsaturated acids.

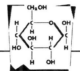

The Chemistry of Nutrition

The term *trans fat* refers to how carbons orient themselves around the double bonds in unsaturated fatty acids. If you were to draw a diagram of a trans-fatty acid, it would look like a straight lineup of carbons. By contrast, another type of unsaturated fat called a *cis* fatty acid has a kink in its chain, causing the chain to bend. Most monounsaturated and polyunsaturated fatty acids in natural fats are in the *cis* form.

Trans Fats and Hydrogenated Fats

Processed foods usually contain a higher proportion of trans fats. Margarine, shortenings, deep-fried foods, baked goods (cakes, brownies, and cookies) mixes, canned soups, and almost all frozen and fast-food restaurant meals are high in trans fats. Animal fats are, in general, also higher than vegetable fats in trans-fatty acids.

Diets with a high proportion of trans fats have been associated with obesity and coronary heart disease. These deleterious effects on health may be because the chemical structure of trans fats is similar to saturated fats, and a diet high in saturated fats is known to increase the risks of heart and blood vessel diseases.

Look for the word *hydrogenated* on the package labels of processed foods. The chemical process of hydrogenation—adding hydrogen atoms all over the place—produces more trans fat in a food.

Hydrogenation is a chemical reaction in which hydrogen atoms attach to the carbons involved in double bonds. The addition of the hydrogens turns the double bond (C=C) into a regular single bond (C-C). With the hydrogens added, the bond looks more like this: -CH-CH-. Hydrogenation thus turns an unsaturated fatty acid into a saturated fatty acid.

The consistency of a fat changes when it becomes hydrogenated. Unsaturated fatty acids are often liquid (oils) at room temperature. The hydrogenation increases the fats' hardness and turns oils into solids. Many oils are sources of unsaturated fats, which are better for you than the solid fats: butter, lard, margarine, and marbling, which are higher in saturated fats.

The wording for hydrogenation can be tricky. A fully hydrogenated fat is the same thing as a saturated fat. Fats labeled "partially hydrogenated" have some single carbon bonds and some double bonds. These foods thus have a mixture of saturated and unsaturated fats. Partially hydrogenated fats also include trans fats, which means they increase the risk of coronary heart disease the same as saturated (fully hydrogenated) fats do.

The Role of Essential Fatty Acids in Health

Linoleic, linolenic, and arachidonic acids are the essential fatty acids (ESAs). They are called essential because the body requires them and they must be supplied in the diet at certain minimum amounts for good nutrition.

Your body can make arachidonic acid from linoleic acid, so enough linoleic acid in the diet may lower your dietary need for arachidonic acid. For this reason, some nutritionists feel that only linoleic and linolenic acids are truly ESAs. In addition, from linolenic acid the body makes two other fatty acids important for good health: docosahexaenoic acid (C22:6) and eicosapentaenoic acid (C20:5).

ESAs play varied roles in the body. They are essential parts of cell membranes, help with vision, enhance nerve and heart function, act as precursors for hormones, and serve in the body's immune system.

Omega Fatty Acids

The ESAs are also referred to as omega fatty acids based on the positioning of the double bonds in the carbon chain. Food products now prominently display *omega* on their package label, and new omega diets have come on the food scene. Increasing the ESAs, or omega-3 and omega-6 fatty acids, in the diet improves overall health. Adequate dietary amounts of these fats are also credited with lowering the risk of coronary heart disease. Dietary ESAs help lower total blood cholesterol levels and promote a healthy ratio of HDL to LDL.

The benefits of omega fatty acids became apparent with research studies in the 1970s showing that Inuit populations have a relatively low incidence of heart diseases despite the high amount of fat in their diet. (The Inuit culture's diet is high in blubber from marine mammals.) Why was the Inuit's high-fat diet seemingly healthy while the American red meat-and-potatoes diet a health disaster? The answer came with the discovery of high levels of omega fatty acids in the fats of marine animals.

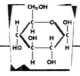

The Chemistry of Nutrition

The essential fatty acids linoleic and linolenic are also sometimes referred to as omega fatty acids. The term *omega* refers to the position of one of the double bonds in the polyunsaturated fatty acid's long chain. Linolenic acid is an omega-3 fatty acid; linoleic acid is an omega-6 fatty acid.

Good sources of omega-3 fatty acids are cold-water fish (tuna, salmon, mackerel, and sardines), walnuts, flaxseed, canola oil, and soybean oil. Good sources of omega-6 fatty acids are chicken, turkey, safflower oil, and corn oil.

Choosing Dietary Fats

Everyone needs fat in their diet because fats and other lipids are essential nutrients. We unfortunately eat too much fat for a variety of reasons. The primary reasons that fat is sometimes out of control in our diets are:

➤ Processed foods and fast foods have a very high content of fats compared with other nutrients.

➤ Restaurant meals are often high in fat because chefs follow the mantra, "Fat is flavor."

➤ Many Americans overeat at every meal and snack between meals. This overeating usually involves taking in excess fat. When you think of a snack, do you think chips, cookies, and ice cream or raw vegetables and fruit? Snacks have a way of undermining otherwise healthy diets.

Here are some tips for putting more good fats in your diet and excluding unhealthy fats:

➤ Increase the proportion of dietary omega fatty acids by eating a serving (3 ounces) of the following two to three times a week: Atlantic salmon, anchovy, sardines, rainbow trout, mackerel, coho salmon, bluefish, striped bass, tuna (white, canned), halibut, or catfish.

➤ Monitor your omega-3 fatty acid intake so within one week it averages 1.6 grams for men and 1.1 grams for women.

➤ Decrease cholesterol intake by decreasing animal fats (beef, organ meats, lard, egg yolks, shrimp, pork, and whole-fat dairy products).

➤ Substitute lean meats and vegetables for red meats and other fatty cuts of meat.

➤ Substitute skim, or fat-free milk, for whole milk and look for 1 percent fat and low-fat dairy products instead of whole-fat products.

➤ Adjust your cholesterol, HDL and LDL, levels by decreasing high-cholesterol foods, increasing high-omega foods, and increasing sources of monounsaturated fatty acids such as olive oil, canola oil, and peanut oil.

➤ Lower your blood levels of trans fats by avoided frozen prepared meals, deep-fried foods, fried fast foods, margarine, and shortening.

➤ Avoid or minimize intake of foods that contain partially hydrogenated fats.

➤ Increase total fiber and whole-grain intake, which helps control calorie and fat intake. Make your diet rich in whole grains, raw vegetables, and fruits.

Nutrition Morsels

Butter seems to have few redeeming qualities in nutrition other than making almost everything taste wonderful. Butter is an animal fat so is high in cholesterol, saturated fats, and trans fats, and low in the good fats that help keep your blood lipids balanced. A tablespoon of butter contains 7.2 grams of saturated fat and 0.3 gram of trans fat. It is a energy-dense food because it delivers no protein, carbohydrates, fiber, or vitamins along with the high-energy fat. But butter is not pure evil. It can be used sparingly to make foods taste good, and keep in mind it contains much less trans fat than margarine (stick) and shortening.

I would not recommend margarine as a healthy substitute for butter. To reduce your butter intake, substitute olive oil for sautéing, other oils (canola, flaxseed, vegetable, and nut) for cooking, all-fruit spreads (no sugar) for toast, and applesauce (no sugar) or hummus for certain baked recipes.

The American Heart Association offers guidelines on managing the amount and types of fats for healthy diets. Begin by limiting the daily amount of saturated fat you eat to less than 7 percent of your total energy intake, limiting trans fats to less than 1 percent of energy, and limiting cholesterol to less than 300 milligrams.

Trying to tackle all of these objectives at once can be difficult and perhaps discouraging. Work out a plan that leads to success by focusing on only one or two of these tips at a time until they become part of your eating habits. Then you can raise the bar by adding more goals for controlling fat intake. Remember that no one is perfect and temptation lurks around every corner, especially corners named birthdays and the holidays. Making a mistake doesn't mean all is lost. Just keep at it as best you can with encouragement from a friend if you need it, or perhaps with help from your doctor or a professional nutritionist.

CHAPTER 13

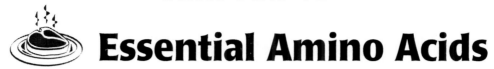

Essential Amino Acids

> ## In This Chapter
>
> ➤ Characteristics of essential and nonessential amino acids
>
> ➤ How amino acids are used to build protein
>
> ➤ Other uses of amino acids by the body
>
> ➤ How we digest and absorb amino acids

In this chapter we turn to amino acids. These are the building blocks of proteins similar to the way glucose is the building block of starch. All proteins are made of amino acids regardless of whether the protein comes from meat or vegetables or is part of your body.

Getting enough protein of good quality into your body is really a case of getting the right amino acids. With a good array and supply of amino acids, your body builds all the proteins that strengthen you, allow you to move, help you reproduce, and enable you to digest your food. If you must go without food for long periods, amino acids help out here too by giving you energy.

What Makes It an Amino Acid?

An amino acid is a fairly simple chemical. All amino acids consist of carbon (C), hydrogen (H), oxygen (O), and nitrogen (N). Some amino acids also contain sulfur.

Almost all amino acids are built on an identical framework made of two carbons, four hydrogens, two oxygens, and one nitrogen. (The exception is the amino acid proline, which consists of carbons connected in a ring structure.) Each amino acid differs from every other amino acid by a side structure that attaches to the standard framework. This appendage, which distinguishes each amino acid in nature, is called an R group.

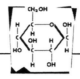

The Chemistry of Nutrition

Amino acids are your primary dietary source of nitrogen. This is a big responsibility because nitrogen-containing chemicals make up about 24 percent of your body. Of all the chemical elements in our diet, nitrogen is often the one at a premium. In other words, carbon, oxygen, and other elements are usually in abundance in the diet but nitrogen is scarcer.

Most amino acids go into making protein, but some of the nitrogen from amino acids gets reassembled into nucleic acids and the auxiliary compounds that participate in energy generation. ATP is one such key energy compound that you cannot live without.

Essential and Nonessential Amino Acids

Nature contains hundreds of amino acids that compose the proteins of animals, plants, and microbes. Your body's proteins can be built using only about twenty different amino acids. Meat is the best source of the specific amino acids you need in your diet. This is because animals have an array of amino acids in their proteins most similar to human proteins.

The twenty amino acids needed by your body can be divided into two types: essential and nonessential. Essential amino acids are those that must be supplied in the diet because your body cannot make them. Nonessential amino acids can be made both by your body and by the bacteria inside your digestive tract (and then absorbed into the bloodstream). The term *nonessential* may be a misnomer; you require both essential and nonessential amino acids to make the proteins that run your body.

Nine amino acids are indispensable in your diet. You must get a steady supply of these amino acids to maintain good health:

> ➤ Histidine

> ➤ Isoleucine

- ➤ Leucine
- ➤ Lysine
- ➤ Methionine
- ➤ Phenylalanine
- ➤ Threonine
- ➤ Tryptophan
- ➤ Valine

Ten amino acids are equally important to you as the essential amino acids, but your body can make these ten nonessential ones, so we worry about them a bit less:

- ➤ Alanine
- ➤ Arginine
- ➤ Asparagine
- ➤ Aspartic acid
- ➤ Cysteine
- ➤ Glutamic acid
- ➤ Glutamine
- ➤ Glycine
- ➤ Proline
- ➤ Serine
- ➤ Tyrosine

When animals (including humans) are young and growing, arginine is an essential amino acid. As an adult, the body makes enough arginine for all protein-building needs. Arginine thus goes from being an essential to a nonessential amino acid.

Nutrition Morsels

Everyone's digestive tract contains hundreds of billions of bacteria. A single gram—about a teaspoon—of intestinal contents holds about a billion bacteria and several thousand protozoa. These microbes take the nitrogen from dietary amino acids and use it to make their own amino acids and proteins.

Some of the amino acids made by the bacteria are useful to the human body, too. When the bacteria die and break apart, we absorb the bacterial amino acids and other things made by these microbes, such as vitamins. In this way the digestive tract's microbes help supply us with a portion of essential nutrients.

How Amino Acids Are Used for Building Protein

Imagine a miniature train made of hundreds of cars. Now in your mind change the train cars into little tin cups. The mouth of each cup has a unique shape.

You are now given a pile of wooden pieces that also differ by shape. Each uniquely shaped piece of wood slips perfectly into a tin cup with a corresponding size and shape. After you have filled each cup, you have in front of you a long strand of wooden pieces in exactly the appropriately shaped cup. Think of this strand as a protein; each piece represents an amino acid. To make a protein exactly the right way, the body must do three things:

1. Make the amino acid strand of the correct length. In other words, some proteins contain exactly 751 amino acids; others contain exactly 4,375, and so on.

2. Put the amino acids in the correct order.

3. Use the correct amino acid at each spot in the train without substituting another incorrect amino acid.

To build protein, your body needs specific amino acids in a specified order. Having five hundred round wooden pieces does you little good if the final tin cup you must fill to complete the train is square. Amino acids in the diet work the same way. An excess of leucine and tryptophan, for instance, cannot help you if you your diet is deficient in lysine.

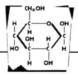

The Chemistry of Nutrition

Of the twenty amino acids we use for making protein, two contain sulfur. These amino acids are methionine and cysteine. Sulfur-containing amino acids are important for protein structure because when they come close to each other in a folded protein, the sulfurs chemically link to each other. This linkage is called a disulfide bond. Disulfide bonds help strengthen various proteins, such as the proteins of feathers and hair. Feather and hair proteins, called keratins, are among the most indestructible proteins in nature.

Once amino acids are put in the right sequence during protein synthesis, the proteins must be folded in a specific way. This folding gives a protein its ability to carry out its functions in the body. Amino acids help in this area, too. When a protein folds up properly, the folding brings certain amino acids closer to each other. These amino acids link up with each other chemically to hold the shape of the folded protein.

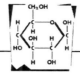

The Chemistry of Nutrition

Amino acids provide the backbone of proteins. Without a protein's proper array and sequence of amino acids plus specific folding, a protein is just a string of amino acids with no purpose. The easiest way to kill a protein's activity is to heat it. When heated, proteins begin to unfold. This unfolding is called denaturation. A denatured protein cannot carry out its normal tasks in the body.

You denature food proteins when you cook your food. Denatured meat proteins become easier to chew and digest. Denatured egg protein congeals from a semisolid to a solid. You can still get all the valuable amino acids you need from denatured protein because the digestive tract breaks down all the protein to absorbable amino acids. After absorbing the amino acids, structures called ribosomes inside your cells begin cranking out long strands of amino acids. An enzyme then folds up the amino acid strand and thereby turns it into one of the hundreds of proteins that keep your metabolism working.

Most of our dietary amino acids end up in muscle, which serves as the body's main protein reserve. The next largest portion is used for making new enzymes and hormones. A small portion of amino acids is burned for energy rather than used for building protein. The remaining amino acids go into the proteins of skin and hair. Unlike muscle, the body cannot recover these amino acids if needed for other jobs. Finally, as much as 12 percent of the protein we eat winds up being unused and the nitrogen is excreted by the kidneys in urine.

How We Digest Amino Acids

Protein digestion begins in the mouth. Saliva contains a variety of protein-degrading enzymes called proteases that start the process of cleaving proteins into smaller pieces. The acids in the stomach help by denaturing food proteins. Finally, proteases of the intestines, made in the pancreas, finish the job of breaking down partially digested protein completely to amino acids.

The cells lining the intestines absorb amino acids in much the same way they absorb sugar. The body uses an interesting mechanism for assuring that amino acids absorbed by the intestines are in about the same amount and variety that the body needs.

In the stomach, the variety of amino acids is about the same as in food protein. Further down the small intestine, however, the variety of amino acids mimics the variety you need for building protein. How does this happen?

The body self-digests a small quantity of cells lining the intestines to release the cells' protein. Digestive enzymes then chew up this protein. Overall, this process helps balance the assortment of amino acids in the intestines. As a result, the amino acids you absorb into your bloodstream are close to the number and proportions that will go into body protein.

What Amino Acids Do in the Body

Amino acids have a surprisingly diverse number of jobs in the body beyond serving as the building blocks of proteins. For example, glutamine has almost twenty different known functions in the body. It works as part of the nervous system, in genetics, as a transporter of nitrogen, as a stimulator of glycogen synthesis, and it even functions in taste.

Other amino acids also serve as vehicles for transporting nitrogen around the body. Many participate in enzyme reactions that generate energy; others act as precursors for compounds that function in immunity. For example, histidine is a precursor for histamine. Histamine is an integral part of your immune response to infections and allergens.

Nutrition Morsels

Many people take amino acid supplements with the hope of boosting their muscle building. The body is designed, however, to get amino acids from food and not supplements that can overwhelm the digestive tract.

Amino acid supplements interfere with the normal activities of intestinal bacteria and likely disrupt overall amino acid absorption. Because some amino acids share the same absorption mechanism, an excess of one amino acid can interfere with the uptake of another amino acid. For example, arginine interferes with lysine uptake and isoleucine interferes with leucine absorption.

Another potential problem comes from an excess of amino acids that can be toxic at high levels in the blood. Methionine, histidine, and cysteine are three known to be dangerous in the body at high levels.

Using Amino Acids for Energy

When a person begins to starve or simply fasts for many hours, the body uses up all available glycogen and fat stores. (Glycogen and adipose tissue rarely decline to zero; a small amount remains even though they cannot be used in metabolism.) After you use up your glycogen and fat, you begin breaking down protein for energy.

Using protein for energy on a consistent basis makes a person lose muscle mass because muscle is where much of the body's protein is stored. In cases of extreme starvation, the body loses almost all its musculature, and the heart weakens. When the body uses protein for energy, the enzymes involved in normal energy generation grab the amino acids as fast as they can. In a desperate attempt to produce ATP to keep the cells alive, amino acids get fed into different energy-generating processes such as glycolysis and the Krebs cycle. Enzymes that run these reactions take the carbons out of the amino acids and discard the rest.

Even though the body uses amino acids for energy in the same reactions it uses sugar, amino acid energy generation is much less efficient. Depleting protein to survive causes the body to lose more heat than normal. In addition, the kidneys must work harder to eliminate the extra nitrogen released when the amino acids get metabolized for energy.

Nutrition Morsels

Three essential amino acids—leucine, isoleucine, and valine—are called branched-chain amino acids (BCAAs) because of their chemical structure. People often take BCAA supplements with their food in the belief that they are giving the body added energy and helping to build muscle. This activity is called an anabolic effect because the BCAAs presumably promote anabolism in the body.

BCAAs might also help energy metabolism, forestall muscle fatigue, and aid the central nervous system (CNS). Doctors prescribe BCAAs for improving appetite in the elderly and for treating CNS diseases such as amyotrophic lateral sclerosis (Lou Gehrig's disease).

But amino acid supplementation can be risky because it causes a dramatic imbalance in the nutrients of a normal diet. BCAAs cause a variety of side effects in metabolism. They should only be used under the direction of a doctor or trained nutritionist.

CHAPTER 14

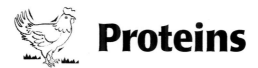 **Proteins**

In This Chapter

➤ Types of animal and plant proteins

➤ Protein quality and balancing amino acids

➤ Protein balance and hazards of high-protein diets

➤ What proteins do in the body

➤ How to boost protein intake the healthy way

In this chapter amino acids work together in teams we know as proteins. Proteins are big molecules. Along with polysaccharides, lipids, and nucleic acids, they are the largest molecules in your cells. These molecules are also among the largest chemicals in your diet. Because your intestines absorb only relatively small chemicals, such as sugars and amino acids, you must break down proteins during digestion. After absorbing the amino acids, your cells build new protein. How do cells do this? By employing yet another specialized type of protein called enzymes.

This chapter explains the importance of proteins in your body and in your diet. Although we cannot say that any one nutrient is more important than the others—you need all nutrients in the proper amounts—it seems hard to conceive of life at all without knowing about protein. It is a major constituent of all cells and the substance most closely associated with the first life on Earth.

Proteins comprise about 15 percent of cells. Proteins vary in size, structure, and composition of amino acids, but all proteins are made of the same six ingredients: carbon (about 53 percent), oxygen (22 percent), nitrogen (17 percent), hydrogen (7 percent), sulfur (1.5 percent), and phosphorus (1 percent). Some proteins contain a small amount of iron. As you can see, proteins serve as a good source of carbon and nitrogen in your diet.

Dietary Protein

Omnivores eat mainly animal and plant proteins. The sources of dietary protein vary in different cultures and geographic regions. In North America, animal sources supply about two-thirds of a person's daily protein intake and plant sources supply the remainder. In other parts of the world, plant protein makes up most of a person's dietary protein. Vegetarians avoid all proteins from animals. Some vegetarians do not eat meat but decide to consume dairy products and eggs. Other vegetarians abstain from these animal sources of proteins, too.

Nutrition Morsels

Fibrous proteins strengthen your body but play few other complicated roles. They offer brute strength and that's about all. By contrast, globular proteins carry out a variety of jobs that keep you alive. Globular proteins react to changing conditions inside and outside the body and help you adjust to these changes. Examples of these versatile proteins are:

➤ Immunoglobulins (also called antibodies): Fight infections

➤ Hemoglobin: Carries oxygen in the bloodstream

➤ Lactoglobulins in milk: Supply protein to newborns

➤ Albumin in egg: A protein source for the embryo

➤ Myoglobin: Stores oxygen in muscle cells

Animal Protein

The previous chapter pointed out that animal proteins give you about the same variety and amount of amino acids needed by your cells to build new protein. Nutritionists therefore say that animal protein is a high-quality protein.

Animal proteins vary widely in how they are constructed and behave in nature. For example, fibrous proteins give the body strength. Proteins such as collagen, elastin, and keratin are almost indestructible and insoluble in water. These proteins strengthen connective tissue, tendons, ligaments, and cartilage as well as hair and skin.

Animal proteins also include water-soluble varieties. Instead of being fibrous, these proteins are called globular proteins. They include enzymes, hormones, hemoglobin, immune system proteins, and components of muscle.

Plant Protein

Plant protein comes mainly from grains and vegetables, and a little bit comes from fruits. (Oils of either vegetable or animal source contain no protein.) Plant proteins often lack the full array of amino acids your body needs. Therefore, if you follow a vegetarian diet, be sure to eat a variety of plant proteins that complement each other in amino acid composition. These are called complementary proteins.

Nutrition Vocabulary

Complementary proteins are proteins that come from two different foods and together supply all nine of the essential amino acids. In a complementary pairing, protein A might supply seven of the essential amino acids but lack sufficient amounts of lysine and methionine. Protein B has a large proportion of these two amino acids. When protein A is eaten with B, a person gets a full supply of amino acids to ensure good nutrition.

Vegetable protein sources are usually divided into legume and nonlegume plants. Legumes are plants that produce seeds in a row inside a pod. The variety of amino acids supplied by legumes usually complements that of nonlegume plants. Therefore, eating a variety of plant proteins to include both legumes and nonlegumes enhances the overall quality of your diet's protein.

Protein Quality

Few proteins, even those from animal sources, supply a perfect variety and amount of the essential amino acids. Good protein nutrition involves eating a variety of protein sources to meet daily needs. A variety of proteins raises your diet's overall protein quality.

Protein quality relates to how well dietary protein supplies the essential amino acids. Animal proteins are generally high-quality protein, and many plant proteins are of poorer quality. When a protein is known to be a good supplier of an amino acid usually low in other sources, this protein becomes valuable to good nutrition.

No protein can supply all the essential amino acids in the perfect proportions you need; one amino acid will always be used up before the others if you depend on just one protein source day in and day out. This first-to-run-out amino acid is called a protein's limiting amino acid.

The concepts of protein quality and limiting amino acids go hand in hand. You can raise your diet's protein quality by knowing the limiting amino acids of common proteins. For example, lysine is a limiting amino acid in wheat and corn. Legumes such as beans, peas, and lentils are good sources of lysine. By adding legumes to your diet, you can fix any lysine deficiencies in your diet.

Limiting Amino Acids

Limiting amino acids are the first amino acids to run out when the body is building new protein. Cells cannot simply skip over that depleted amino acid and make a plan B version of a protein. Instead, when the limiting amino acid is no longer available, cells stop making the protein. This can have serious consequences if the protein you need is a vital enzyme or an antibody or hemoglobin!

Vegetarians usually must pay special attention to the limiting amino acids of food proteins. Because plant proteins are generally of poorer quality than animal proteins, selecting a variety of complementary plant proteins help raise the diet's protein quality. Complementary proteins lessen the risk of amino acid limitation.

Amino Acid Score

Figuring out the exact limiting amino acids in your diet can be tricky. You have no way of knowing which amino acid in your body is about to run out first when your cells gear up to make new muscle, a hormone, enzymes, or other proteins. Nutritionists therefore assign a score, called the amino acid score, to many food proteins to help you select proteins of the highest quality and digestibility. On the 0.0 to 1.0 scale, higher-quality proteins approach 1.0 and lower-quality proteins are nearer 0.0:

> ➤ Egg white (ovalbumin): 1.0
> ➤ Milk (casein): 1.0
> ➤ Milk (whey): 1.0
> ➤ Soybeans: 1.0
> ➤ Beef: 0.92–1.0
> ➤ Black beans (dry): 0.75
> ➤ Rice: 0.62–0.65
> ➤ Peanuts: 0.52
> ➤ Corn: 0.35–0.47
> ➤ Wheat (gluten): 0.25–0.37

Nutrition Morsels

The amino acid score is a numerical value that ranks all food proteins on a scale from 0.0 to 1.0. Some nutrition resources use an equivalent 0–100 scale. The score's full name is the Protein Digestibility-Corrected Amino Acid Score (PDCAAS) because it considers both the variety of essential amino acids in a protein and the body's ability to digest the protein. After all, a protein of superior quality is not much use to you if your body cannot digest it. The World Health Organization (WHO) first proposed the use of the PDCAAS to help professional nutritionists formulate diets in parts of the world where food selection is limited and many children and adults are malnourished.

Complete Protein and Incomplete Protein

To avoid discussing proteins in terms of a numerical amino acid score, some nutritionists use two terms that make it easy for you to guess a protein's quality: complete and incomplete protein.

➤ Complete protein contains ample amounts of all the essential amino acids.

➤ Incomplete protein lacks one or more essential amino acids.

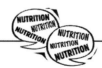

Nutrition Vocabulary

Casein and whey are both proteins of milk. When all the cream (fat portion) has been removed from milk, the result is skim (or skimmed) milk, which contains water, lactose, and the proteins casein and whey. If a food chemist wanted to recover only the milk's whey proteins, the chemist would remove the casein by centrifugation. Casein and whey proteins are often sold separately as dietary protein supplements.

As you've learned earlier, even a complete protein with a high amino acid score has at least one limiting amino acid. Eating a variety of protein foods helps you take in sufficient amounts of all amino acids. To do this, eat a variety of as many of these foods as you can:

➤ Lean meats (chicken, pork, and lean red meat)

➤ Fish and shellfish

➤ Milk and yogurt (both fat-free) and cheese

➤ Egg whites

➤ Legumes

Protein Balance

Protein balance is a state of your body in which you are either adding protein or losing it. People who are adding protein are in a positive protein balance. Positive balance occurs in growing children or when an adult is recovering from an injury or illness, building muscle (such as in weight training), or carrying a fetus.

Negative protein balance occurs when the body loses protein. The reasons for negative balance include starvation, prolonged fasting, some acute illnesses, and advanced age.

When a person takes in about the same amount of protein as is normally lost by the body, this state is called protein equilibrium.

The exact protein needs for a person are difficult to determine. Your individual protein needs depend on your overall health, age, level of physical activity, and hormones.

Nutritionists advise that healthy adults get 0.8 grams of protein per kilogram of body weight to maintain protein equilibrium. (That equals about 1.76 grams of protein per pound of body weight or 56 grams of protein for a 156-pound person.) The following formula helps you calculate your estimated protein needs:

(Weight in pounds) X (0.454) X (0.8) = grams of dietary protein

Nutrition Morsels

Do you know what red meat is? You probably think of red meat as steaks, chops (including pork), and hamburger. These red meats are major dietary sources of fat (trans and saturated), calories, and cholesterol. They also offer benefits such as high-quality protein, many B vitamins, some minerals, and energy. When watching your total red meat intake, don't forget about the other food sources of red meat. Eating sausages, hotdogs, deli meats (cold cuts), stews, ham, and bacon boosts your total red meat intake.

High-Protein Diets

Many athletes and people trying to lose weight have become advocates of high-protein diets. Indeed, diets that give you a positive protein balance can help build muscle and will likely help to shed pounds. High-protein diets can help in weight loss because the space taken up in the diet by fat-producing carbohydrates and fats are replaced with protein, which the body does not turn into fat. But high-protein diets might lead to other health problems ranging from minor to life-threatening. Here are some things to consider if you are wondering about the consequences of a high-protein diet:

➤ Extra dietary protein puts an added burden on the kidneys because you must excrete excess nitrogen as urea.

➤ High intake of animal proteins may contribute to kidney stones.

➤ High intake of red meats is associated with a higher risk for cardiovascular disease and colon cancer.

➤ High intake of red meats and shellfish may increase fat intake and lead to weight gain.

➤ Increased protein intake usually causes a lowered intake of fiber, some vitamins, and some minerals.

➤ Lots of protein and less fiber and carbohydrates in the diet can cause dehydration and bad breath!

Some high-protein diets have become popular as a fast approach to weight loss. But many nutritionists think of these diets as fads that lead to other nutritional problems. When you are in doubt about a new type of diet being popularized, try to remember that good nutrition always relates to a good balance of nutrients. Promoting one nutrient over all the others is never a safe path to health.

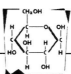

The Chemistry of Nutrition

Urea is a simple chemical made in the kidneys as a way to get excess nitrogen out of the body. Marine animals can excrete nitrogen as ammonia, but ammonia is toxic and would irritate land animals if we were forced to store it in our body until we could get rid of it. The kidneys solve this problem by hooking two ammonia molecules together to make urea, which dissolves in water and is much less irritating to tissues than ammonia. Urea makes up more than 50 percent of the substances dissolved in urine. Although this is an easy way for us to excrete excess nitrogen, we must remember to replace the large amounts of water we lose with urinary excretion.

Insects, land snails, reptiles, and birds excrete nitrogen in uric acid rather than urea. Like urea, uric acid is not toxic, but it is insoluble in water. These animals excrete the solid chemical without losing much of the body's water.

What Proteins Do in the Body

Proteins cover so many responsibilities in your body that I could hardly sum up their importance in one sentence. Biologists tend to group proteins into big classes based on their general role in cells or in the body. By classifying proteins this way, you can learn about them as part of eight major groups. Each of the following groups can contain, however, several to hundreds of individual proteins with narrowly defined jobs:

1. Enzymes: Proteins that run chemical reactions inside cells, in tissue, blood, and the digestive tract.

2. Structural proteins: The fibers that support the body, such as those found in connective tissue, as well as the protein (keratin) of skin, hair, fur, feathers, horns, claws, and nails.

3. Transport proteins: Proteins that help nutrients get into cells or that carry substances through the bloodstream; for example, hemoglobin, which carries oxygen.

4. Hormones: Some hormones, such as insulin, are proteins. Other protein hormones are glucagon, prolactin, and growth hormone.

5. Contractile proteins: Mainly actin and myosin, these proteins give the body movement by moving muscles. The proteins that control cilia and flagella also belong to this group.

6. Antibodies: Proteins that help defend the body against invasion (or infection) from foreign matter.

7. Receptors: Proteins on the outside of nerve and other cells that help in cell-to-cell communication.

8. Storage proteins: These store amino acids for special purposes, such as for embryos (egg whites and seeds) or the newborn (milk proteins).

Enzymes

Enzymes are the body's catalysts. This means they help chemical reactions go forward in the body without using up much energy. Without enzymes, many chemical reactions would require a huge input of energy to turn chemical A into product B. In chemical manufacturing plants, this energy is often supplied in the form of very high heat. Since your body is not set up to act as a blast furnace, enzymes play a vital role in turning A into B without demanding high temperatures. Many enzymes need only a small input of ATP, which you supply through respiration.

Like all proteins, enzymes contain a specific assortment of amino acids lined up in a particular order. The enzyme is folded up in a very specific pattern. Every enzyme contains a section of amino acids, often located at a particular fold, that connects with a chemical to be converted into something else. The chemical acted on by an enzyme is called a substrate. Every enzyme in nature has at least one substrate and a product. For example, the first step in glycolysis is the attachment of a phosphate to glucose. The enzyme hexokinase does this attachment. Thus, glucose is hexokinase's substrate and a chemical called glucose-6-phosphate is hexokinase's product.

Fortunately, enzymes work without your need to think about which ones are required and when, and turning them on and off. Your only job to keep them all working properly is to eat enough proteins, carbohydrates, some fat, and vitamins and minerals.

Boosting Protein Intake

Most people living in North America and other wealthy western societies get enough protein. The average North American man consumes about 100 grams of protein daily, and women consume about 65 grams daily. Only people who have endured long illnesses, severe injury, malnutrition, or other events leading to prolonged negative protein balance should boost their protein intake.

Boosting your protein intake is best done by following these guidelines:

➤ Eat a varied diet of protein sources plus carbohydrates, fats, vitamins, and minerals to assure adequate energy supply.

➤ Stay hydrated because your enzymes need water to run protein-building and storage reactions.

➤ Consume a variety of protein sources to assure adequate intake of all the essential amino acids.

➤ Avoid amino acid supplements because these can lead to amino acid imbalance.

➤ Target the recommended daily protein intake levels rather than high-protein diets that supply excessive amounts of protein.

PART FOUR

Vitamins, Minerals, Salt, and Water

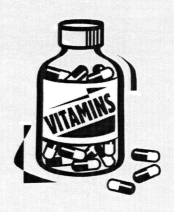

CHAPTER 15

 # Water-Soluble Vitamins: B Vitamins and Vitamin C

> ## In This Chapter
>
> ➤ Introduction to water-soluble vitamins
>
> ➤ The uses and sources of B vitamins and vitamin C
>
> ➤ Overview of water-soluble vitamin deficiencies

In this chapter you embark on the nitty-gritty of nutrition: the vitamins. Unlike carbohydrates, fats, and proteins, vitamins are needed by the body in very small, and sometimes very specific, amounts. We know vitamins are good for us but sometimes people make a mistake when considering vitamins, assuming that if a little is good, a lot is better. Nothing could be further from the truth! Like all nutrients, the body needs what it needs and doesn't want any extra amounts floating around.

This chapter introduces you to the vitamins that dissolve in water. These water-soluble vitamins are the B vitamins and vitamin C. You will learn to distinguish between these vitamins, where the body uses them, and how the body deals with excess amounts of these vitamins. Finally, each section also summarizes the consequences of not getting enough of a particular water-soluble vitamin.

An Introduction to Vitamins

A vitamin is a compound needed by the body in small amounts, and is supplied by the diet in small amounts to run chemical reactions. Nutritionists divide vitamins into two groups

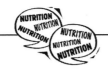

Nutrition Vocabulary

A coenzyme is a chemical that combines with an inactive enzyme to make the enzyme active in the body.

based on their solubility in water: water-soluble and fat-soluble. The B vitamins and vitamin C are water-soluble. Fat-soluble vitamins are A, D, E, and K.

Vitamins are essential in the diet because the body cannot make them in amounts needed for normal metabolism. In metabolism, vitamins serve as coenzymes, which are substances that help enzymes work.

Vitamins vary in chemical structure, but they all have two things in common:

1. The body does not make enough of them to maintain health.

2. When a vitamin is absent from the diet, health declines.

When the diet does not supply a vitamin in the amounts needed by the body, the result can be poor overall health or a defined disease with known symptoms called a vitamin deficiency disease. Many of the functions we now know belong to vitamins were discovered by studying deficiency diseases.

Vitamins can be supplied by the diet or in supplements. Vitamin supplements often provide vitamin amounts called megadoses that are much larger than those normally found in the diet.

Nutrition Morsels

A megadose is the intake of any nutrient in amounts much higher than needed to prevent deficiency. Some vitamin supplements have amounts two to ten times higher than would be found in a normal balanced diet. Such megadoses can be dangerous to health. They should not be taken without advice from a physician or trained nutritionist. When prescribed by a professional, these vitamin doses are called pharmacological dose.

Where Water-Soluble Vitamins Come From

All vitamins come from plant and animal foods as well as the synthesized forms made in laboratories. With few exceptions, synthetic vitamins work the same in the body as natural vitamins from food.

Most water-soluble vitamins are not stored in the body and so must be part of your daily food intake. The body can store vitamins B6 and B12 slightly better than other water-soluble vitamins.

In general, grains, vitamin-fortified cereals, and meats are good sources of B vitamins. Usually, a good source of one B vitamin is also a good source of all the others. Fresh fruit and vegetables are good sources of vitamin C.

Nutrition Morsels

The B vitamins were originally thought to be a single vitamin. As scientists learned more about the chemistry of nutrition, they discovered what they thought was vitamin B was actually a group of distinct chemicals. Each newly identified vitamin in this so-called B complex received a number from 1 through 12. Thus, thiamin became known as B1, B-1, or B_1. With more studies, nutritionists learned that four of the numbered chemicals had no role in the body's metabolism. These four compounds were deleted from the list of B vitamins and today we have no vitamins B4, B8, B10, or B11.

B Vitamins

Eight B vitamins exist. They are all coenzymes important in energy metabolism. A ninth compound called choline is similar to B vitamins but has not been classified as a vitamin. This is because nutrition researchers have not yet determined if choline is essential in human diets.

Vitamin B1: Thiamin

Most North American diets contain sufficient thiamin. Like most B vitamins, it has more than one role in the body, but its most important job is in energy metabolism. Thiamin works steps that burn carbohydrates and amino acids for energy.

The recommended daily intake for thiamin for adults is 1.1–1.2 milligrams. (Men usually require the higher level for this and the other B vitamins.) The best food sources for thiamin are pork products (ham and Canadian bacon), whole grains such as wheat germ, enriched or fortified cereals, and particular vegetables such as potatoes, acorn squash, and green beans. Rice is a poor source of thiamin unless the package is labeled Enriched.

A deficiency of thiamin in the diet lasting for more than ten days leads to the disease beriberi. The symptoms are weakness and poor coordination in arms and legs, loss of appetite, irritability, and a nervous tingling sensation. Prolonged thiamin deficiency leads to more serious nervous system disorders and possible heart failure.

Nutrition Vocabulary

Fortified and enriched food products have had extra vitamins added to them during manufacturing. Fortified foods contain extra vitamins and minerals in addition to the natural amounts already in the food. By contrast, enriched foods contain nutrients that have been added because the natural food lacks these substances.

Vitamin B2: Riboflavin

Riboflavin is integral in energy release from foods, particularly fats. Riboflavin also helps other vitamins and minerals work in the body and is one of several nutrients that act as antioxidants, chemicals that protect cells against the harmful effects of oxygen.

The recommended daily intake of riboflavin for adults is 1.1–1.3 milligrams. The best foods for supplying riboflavin are milk and milk products, enriched grains and cereals, meat, eggs, fish (especially oysters), and green vegetables such as asparagus, broccoli, and spinach. Dairy products are the main source of riboflavin in North American diets.

Riboflavin deficiency is a health problem in many regions outside the United States. After two months on a riboflavin-deficient diet, people may experience these symptoms:

➤ Inflammation of the mouth and tongue

➤ Irritated and dry, cracking skin, especially at the corners of the mouth

➤ Eye disorders

➤ Increased sensitivity to sunlight

Vitamin B3: Niacin

Niacin works in the enzyme steps that get energy from glucose during respiration. In the body, niacin occurs only as part of two coenzymes: nicotinic acid and nicotinamide. These two compounds are also crucial in the steps used to build new cell constituents.

The body can make about 50 percent of needed niacin from the amino acid tryptophan. But many people also need 14–16 milligrams of dietary niacin daily, so nutritionists view niacin as an essential nutrient.

Poultry and beef, enriched cereals, wheat bran, fish (especially tuna and salmon), peanuts, and asparagus supply good amounts of niacin.

Almost every metabolic process in the body uses niacin, so a deficiency of this vitamin happens quickly and is serious. Niacin deficiency disease is called pellagra, which in Greek means rough skin. In addition to dermatitis on skin exposed to sunlight, pellagra includes weakness, weight loss, diarrhea, and progression to dementia.

Vitamin B5: Pantothenic Acid

Pantothenic acid makes up part of coenzyme A, which is central to the energy-generating steps of burning carbohydrates, fats, and proteins.

Pantothenic acid is widespread in foods so it is almost impossible to be deficient in this vitamin when eating a balanced diet. Good sources are milk and milk products, eggs, mushrooms, peanuts, meat, sunflower seeds, and many vegetables. The word *pantothenic* is from the Greek language for "from everywhere." Adults should get about 5 milligrams of this vitamin a day; most people probably consume more.

Vitamin B6: Pyridoxine

Vitamin B6 is actually a group of three coenzymes involved in carbohydrate, fat, and protein metabolism. When added to foods, it is often called pyridoxine.

Vitamin B6 is especially important in the steps of amino acid use and assembly into proteins. The body also uses this vitamin to make neurotransmitters, which are chemicals that carry impulses between adjacent nerve fibers. Last but not least, vitamin B6 is necessary for hemoglobin production and the manufacture of new white blood cells. Since white blood cells are needed for healthy immunity, vitamin B6 is particularly important in fighting infections.

A wide variety of foods supply the needed amounts (1.3–1.7 milligrams daily) of vitamin B6:

- ➤ Fish
- ➤ Meat
- ➤ Dairy products
- ➤ Enriched or fortified cereals

➤ Wheat germ

➤ Vegetables and fruits such as potatoes, spinach, cauliflower, avocados, bananas, dates, and cantaloupe

Vitamin B6 deficiency is rare. Symptoms may include nausea and nervous disorders. People most susceptible to B6 deficiency are highly trained athletes, pregnant women, and alcohol abusers.

Vitamin B7: Vitamin H, or Biotin

This vitamin goes by many names but is usually known as biotin. Biotin serves mainly as a carrier of carbon when your cells make new carbohydrates and fat or when you need to burn amino acids for energy.

The recommended daily intake for biotin is about 30 milligrams for adults. Most diets supply biotin in ample amounts. Foods such as peanut butter, egg yolks, cheese, and cauliflower are good sources. If you like dishes using raw eggs, beware. The protein avidin in raw egg whites interferes with biotin absorption. Cooking eggs denatures avidin and makes biotin available for use by your body.

Biotin deficiency is noticeable as scaly, inflamed skin, appetite loss, nausea, vomiting, anemia, and muscle weakness and pain. The onset of these symptoms varies from person to person because the bacteria of the digestive tract may provide some of your biotin needs.

Vitamin B9: Folic Acid

No one ever calls this vitamin B9; it almost always goes by the name folic acid or folate.

Folate is a carbon carrier in cells and is essential for building DNA and metabolizing various amino acids. A folate deficiency mostly affects new, growing cells because normal DNA synthesis has been disrupted. For example, when it is time for bone marrow to make new red blood cells (RBCs), insufficient amounts of DNA cannot sustain the two new cells that should arise from a dividing parent cell. As a result, cells stall in an immature form called a megaloblast. A megaloblast is an oversized RBC that cannot carry as much oxygen as a normal cell. The condition is known as megaloblastic anemia and can develop after about ten weeks on a folate-deficient diet.

About 10 percent of people in North America have a genetic disorder that also affects folate metabolism. Symptoms of folate deficiency include tongue inflammation, diarrhea, depression, mental confusion, and other problems in nerve function in addition to anemia.

Good folate foods are green, leafy vegetables (spinach, asparagus, Romaine lettuce, sprouts, and broccoli), dried beans (especially lentils), organ meats, and orange juice. The recommended daily intake for folate for adults is about 400 micrograms. (A microgram is 0.001 of a milligram.)

Vitamin B12: Cobalamin

Vitamin B12 offers an excellent example of how vitamins and minerals work together and how you depend on the bacteria of your digestive tract for good health. Vitamin B12 can work in the body only if it forms a complex around the mineral cobalt. (It is sometimes called cyanocobalamin for the blue tint given the vitamin by cobalt; *cyano* refers to the color blue.) Thus, one of the important nutritional purposes of cobalt is to help vitamin B12 work. The bacteria of the digestive tract also need cobalt to make their own B12. Humans get some of their B12 needs by absorbing this bacterial vitamin from the intestines.

Vitamin B12 deficiency usually arises from an inability to absorb this large compound rather than from dietary deficiencies. It is one of the largest compounds our cells must absorb. Doctors can prescribe vitamin B12 injections for people with absorption problems, especially the elderly. The progressive decline in B12 absorption leads to a condition called pernicious anemia. It is termed *pernicious* because the condition is associated with destruction of systems, especially the nervous system.

B12 has varied functions in the body, mainly as a coenzyme in carbon metabolism, especially folate and amino acid reactions. Folate cannot function unless vitamin B12 is also at adequate levels. Thus, B12 deficiency sometimes gives the symptoms of folate deficiency.

Nutrition Morsels

Choline is a vitamin-like compound. Some nutritionists classify choline with the B vitamins because of its similar role in metabolism and nerve function. Choline is part of the chemical acetylcholine, which is a neurotransmitter. This chemical enables nerves to control muscles and also helps with brain function, mainly in the areas of attention, memory, and learning. Choline also helps make up the cell membrane as part of lecithin. Choline is widespread in many foods.

Other vitamin-like compounds are:

➤ Inositol: A is part of cell membranes

➤ Taurine: A component of bile salts

➤ Carnitine: A compound that aids energy-release from fatty acids

➤ Lipoic acid: An antioxidant that helps key steps in carbohydrate metabolism

Although other vitamin-like compounds have drawn attention over the years (coenzyme Q or coQ; vitamin B17 or laetrile; vitamin Bt or carnitine; and vitamin B13 or orotic acid), nutritionists believe that all the essential B vitamins have been discovered and no unknown essential ones have eluded us.

Another effect of B12 deficiency is damage to muscle fibers, leading to paralysis. Specifically, B12-deficient people cannot form strong myelin sheaths. Myelin sheaths cover and insulate nerve fibers. The destruction of this covering has devastating effects on nerve function and can lead to death.

Microbes are the only known natural source of vitamin B12. Animal foods are therefore sources of the vitamin because animals also have large populations of microbes in their gut. For B12, eat foods such as meat, organ meats (liver, kidneys, and heart), milk, seafood, and eggs. Many breakfast cereals are enriched with B12. Nutritionists recommend adults get 2.4 micrograms of vitamin B12 daily.

Vitamin C: Ascorbic Acid

Most animals make their own vitamin C, but not humans. Humans must consume from 30 to 180 milligrams vitamin C daily, and they absorb only 80 percent of it. You cannot solve this dilemma by taking megadoses of vitamin C; high C intake further decreases its absorption. Fortunately, vitamin C is abundant in plenty of foods. The best sources are citrus fruits, broccoli, brussels sprouts, cauliflower, red and green peppers, tomato juice, strawberries, papaya, and kiwi fruit.

Vitamin C has five major functions in the body:

1. Antioxidant activity: The vitamin easily reacts with oxygen, sparing the destructive effects of oxygen on other cellular compounds.

2. Collagen synthesis: Vitamin C helps strengthen collagen during this protein's synthesis. The term *limeys* refers to eighteenth-century British sailors who sucked on citrus fruits to ward off the vitamin deficiency known as scurvy. Scurvy is characterized by skin, bone, and other connective tissue injuries due to improper collagen formation.

3. Iron absorption: Vitamin C helps the intestinal lining absorb iron. It also helps in the functioning of certain iron-containing enzymes.

4. Enzyme activity: Vitamin C plays specific roles in helping certain copper-containing enzymes to work.

5. Immune activity: Vitamin C plays roles in immunity. Certain immune system cells rely on the vitamin for full activity, and vitamin C mediates histamine levels. Histamine is one of the immune substances that jumps into action in the early stages of infection. It also causes many of the uncomfortable symptoms of colds and allergies.

Vitamin C Excess

Megadoses of vitamin C open you to the risk of a disease called rebound scurvy. High doses of C cause the body to make more vitamin C-metabolizing enzymes. When you stop taking the megadose, those enzymes keep working and chew up any vitamin C even if you take the vitamin at normal levels. As a result, rebound scurvy leads to the same health risks as regular scurvy.

Nutrition Morsels

Biochemist Linus Pauling proposed in 1970 that megadoses (1 gram daily) of vitamin C could fight colds. His book, *Vitamin C and the Common Cold*, sold millions and perhaps influenced millions of people to take large doses of vitamin C at the first sign of a cold. Many studies have since been conducted to substantiate or perhaps disprove Pauling's theory. Pauling's critics have pointed out that the scientific evidence behind his ideas on vitamin C was thin. No body of evidence has accumulated to prove that vitamin C megadoses are effective in fighting the common cold.

How We Digest Water-Soluble Vitamins

Any coenzyme complexes of the B vitamins in food get broken down to the bare vitamin in the intestines. The body then absorbs the simple form of the vitamin before reassembling it into its coenzyme form.

For most dietary B vitamins and vitamin C, 50–90 percent of the vitamin is absorbable. This high absorption capability means that these vitamins have high bioavailability.

Only vitamin B12 requires extra effort to absorb. To protect B12 from being destroyed by stomach acids, the vitamin must first bind with a protein from saliva. After making it past this harsh environment of the stomach, B12 must detach from the saliva protein and connect with another protein called intrinsic factor. Intrinsic factor helps the large intestine absorb both dietary B12 and the B12 made by intestinal bacteria. Even then, nutritionists calculate that a person normally absorbs only half of the B12 in the large intestine.

How the Body Manages Water-Soluble Vitamins

As you might guess, water is a vital part of water-soluble vitamin metabolism. These vitamins need ample water intake for three reasons:

1. Vitamin absorption requires water to be present in the intestines.

2. The body's chemical reactions that involve B vitamins and vitamin C all need water.

3. Excess water-soluble vitamins must be flushed from the body and this requires healthy kidneys and adequate water intake.

Only vitamins B6 and B12 are stored in the body for extended periods.

Unless you have adopted a diet that is drastically out of balance, you should have no problems with the water-soluble vitamins throughout your life. The only exception may be vitamin B12, which sometimes needs extra monitoring to ensure you receive adequate levels.

CHAPTER 16

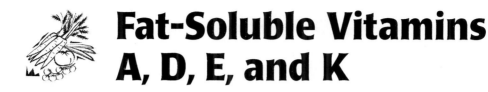

Fat-Soluble Vitamins A, D, E, and K

In This Chapter

➤ The difference between fat- and water-soluble vitamins

➤ Roles and dietary requirements of fat-soluble vitamins

➤ Deficiency and toxicity symptoms of fat-soluble vitamins

In this chapter you will learn about the vitamins that cannot dissolve in water, the fat-soluble vitamins. Because three of these four vitamins (A, D, and E) hide in fat, they can stay in the body much longer than the water-soluble vitamins. Fat-soluble vitamins can even accumulate in the body. For this reason, you must take extra care in watching your intake of fat-soluble vitamin sources, whether the vitamins come in the form of food or a pill. The safest way to manage your vitamin intake is to eat a variety of foods known to be good sources of vitamins and minerals as well as carbohydrates, fats, and proteins.

How Fat-Soluble Vitamins Differ from Water-Soluble Vitamins

Because fat-soluble vitamins can accumulate in the body, they can lead to toxic effects more readily than water-soluble vitamins. Megadoses of fat-soluble vitamins are therefore a much greater health concern than megadoses of water-soluble vitamins.

In general, fat-soluble vitamins withstand heat, cooking, freezing, and storage a bit better than water-soluble vitamins, which can be destroyed by long, improper storage. While water-soluble vitamins can be lost if foods are overcooked, cooked in water, or exposed to air for long periods, fat-soluble vitamins hide in the fatty portions of food and stay relatively protected. Vitamin E is an exception. It can be destroyed by light, oxygen, metals, and deep-fat frying.

Nutrition Morsels

Multivitamin supplements or one-a-day vitamins contain a mixture of vitamins and usually include a variety of essential minerals. For safe use of multivitamin supplements, make sure they contain no more than two times the recommended daily dose of vitamins, particularly fat-soluble vitamins, for adults. This is especially true for vitamin A, which accumulates to toxic levels in the body with prolonged intake of high doses.

Vitamin A

Vitamin A was the first vitamin discovered, and it was discovered in the early 1900s. It has several well-studied functions and a few roles that have been discovered only recently. The three well-known functions are:

1. Vision: A form of the vitamin called retinal helps the eyes adjust to bright and dim light. One of the first signs of vitamin A deficiency is a lessening of this adjustment called night blindness.

2. Antioxidant: A precursor to vitamin A called carotenes scavenges low levels of oxygen in tissues, thereby protecting cells against oxygen toxicity. As an antioxidant, vitamin A is believed to have beneficial effects in preventing cardiovascular disease and cancer. Both of these roles, however, need more study.

3. Cell differentiation: Vitamin A participates in complex steps that begin with cell differentiation in a fetus and continue through the newborn's growth. The vitamin is known to interact with DNA and the movement of information from genes to proteins (called gene expression). Vitamin A also aids the development of white blood cells and helps cell-to-cell communication in the body.

Retinoids and Carotenoids

Vitamin A occurs in food in various forms and also works in the body in different forms. Retinoids are preformed versions of the vitamin. (Retinol is another name for vitamin A.) They are found naturally in food, mainly foods from animal sources. Retinoids are also used as topical applicants for skin, due to their antioxidant activities and other potential benefits to maintaining healthy skin.

Some of the common retinoids you might hear about in nutrition or in cosmetics and skin care are:

> ➤ Retinol: This is the natural form of vitamin A. The body converts retinol to active forms that help with vision, cell reproduction, and other functions.

> ➤ Retinal: Also called retinaldehyde, this is the form of vitamin A that helps with proper vision and cell differentiation in the body. The specific form of retinal that aids low-light vision is 11-cis-retinal. In the eye it combines with a protein called opsin to form rhodopsin. Rhodopsin is a light-sensitive compound that gives you your vision.

> ➤ Retinoic acid: This form of vitamin A acts mainly in cell development and growth.

Carotenoids are a group of compounds in nature that serve as precursors to vitamin A. Another word for a vitamin precursor is *provitamin*. In other words, after digesting a carotenoid, the body can convert certain carotenoids to vitamin A. Of the roughly six hundred carotenoids known in nature, about fifty can be converted to vitamin A.

Because of provitamin-to-vitamin conversion, nutritionists view the good food sources of carotenoids as also good sources of the vitamin. Some of the best carotenoid sources are spinach, kale, collard greens, carrots, sweet potatoes, acorn squash, and mangoes.

Carotenoids are pigments that give foods, mainly vegetables, a color. They range from yellow to orange to red, so selecting fruits or vegetables of these colors is a good way to ensure you get enough dietary vitamin A. In addition to being a precursor to forming vitamin A in the body, carotenoids also act as antioxidants. They may play additional supportive roles in a variety of other body activities such as immunity, reproduction, bone development, and skin function.

Some of the carotenoids that act as provitamins in human nutrition are:

> ➤ Beta-carotene, or β-carotene: The principal carotene of our diet. To make vitamin A, the body splits β-carotene into two equal pieces. Each piece gives rise to a molecule of vitamin A.

➤ Alpha-carotene, or α-carotene: The chemical structure of this carotene is almost identical to the beta form, and it works the same way in the body.

➤ β-cryptoxanthin: Similar in chemical structure to the red-orange carotenes, this pigment belongs to a larger class of yellow pigments called xanthophylls.

Other carotenoids are usually present in your diet if you eat lots of fruits and vegetables, but the body cannot turn most of these pigments into vitamin A. So if a product touts itself as being a good source of carotenoids, be sure to look specifically for the carotenes or β-cryptoxanthin on the food label. Some carotenoids with little value as a provitamin are lutein, lycopene, and zeaxanthin.

Vitamin A Requirements

Adults need enough vitamin A or carotenoids in their diet to supply 700–900 micrograms of the vitamin. Food labels state 1,000 micrograms or 5,000 IU (international units) as a daily recommended amount for adults.

Dark green vegetables and yellow-orange vegetables and fruits are good sources of carotenoids. Good sources of the preformed vitamin are liver, fish, fish oils, eggs, and dairy products fortified with vitamins.

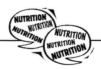

Nutrition Vocabulary

The international unit, or IU, is an approximate value for telling you how much vitamin a food or vitamin supplement provides. IU values for fat-soluble vitamins were established for humans decades ago based on feeding studies in animals. Today, nutritionists tend to prefer using milligrams or micrograms for describing a vitamin requirement.

Vitamin A Deficiency and Toxicity

Vitamin A deficiency is rare in developed countries. In fact, toxicity from getting too much of the vitamin may be more common in North America.

The main deficiency conditions are night blindness, xerophthalmia (called dry eye, the inability to produce sufficient mucus in the eye), and age-related macular degeneration. In poor countries where malnutrition is common, vitamin A deficiency is a major cause of blindness.

Too much vitamin A (not carotenoids) intake shows up first as an orange coloring of the skin, starting in the fingertips, and severe headache. Hair loss and vomiting follow, and then liver damage occurs. As the liver becomes overloaded with excess vitamin A it cannot clear from the body, toxicity spreads to the central nervous system, bones, and skin. These problems begin after several weeks of vitamin A intake exceeding about 8 milligrams per day. Specific effects are:

➤ Increased pressure in cerebral spinal fluid, causing headaches, nausea, anorexia (loss of appetite), and ataxia (loss of muscle coordination)

➤ Joint pain

➤ Alopecia (hair loss)

➤ Drying and scaling of skin

Possible toxicity from high vitamin A intake is of special concern to pregnant women. Too much vitamin A in the early months of pregnancy can cause malformation of the growing fetus.

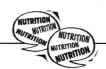

Nutrition Vocabulary

Provitamins are substances that the body can convert into an active vitamin, if needed. Thus, a provitamin means the same as a vitamin precursor.

Vitamin D

Vitamin D behaves as a hormone in the body. It controls intestinal absorption of calcium, calcium movement into and out of bone, and calcium reabsorption by the kidneys. Overall, it works with other hormones to regulate calcium movement in the body and bone health. Vitamin D also helps out in the development of certain types of tissue. This vitamin is important in development of the skin, ovaries, prostate, and breast tissue.

The body can make its own vitamin D. Some nutritionists feel vitamin D is not an essential nutrient at all in people who can supply 100 percent of their own vitamin D needs. We begin the steps toward making vitamin D when the skin is exposed to sunlight. The sun's ultraviolet (UV) light converts a cholesterol-based compound in the skin called 7-dehydrocholesterol, to vitamin D3 (also called cholecalciferol). This material travels in blood to the liver and kidneys, which convert it again to the active form of the vitamin.

We need a specific type of UV light called UVB to start the vitamin D process in the skin. UVB light is most intense in most parts of North America between 9 am and 4 pm. The use of sunscreens above SPF 8 decreases your ability to produce vitamin D.

Vitamin D Requirements

Adults should consume about 5 micrograms (200 IU) of vitamin D per day to supplement whatever vitamin the body produces. Food labels usually cite 10 micrograms per day as the daily adult requirement.

You can meet your vitamin D requirements by getting moderate sun exposure. Too much sunlight exposure causes other serious health problems, such as skin cancer. Fortunately, a variety of foods are good sources of preformed vitamin D. The best foods are fatty fish, such as salmon, tuna, and sardines; vitamin D-fortified milk; and fortified breakfast cereals.

Vitamin D Deficiency and Toxicity

Vitamin D deficiency is rare in adults living in North America and other industrialized places. The highest risk for deficiency occurs in infants and toddlers in northern latitudes, where sunlight exposure is minimal. The deficiency, which can lead to the disease rickets, keeps a child's long leg bones from developing normally and leads to bowed legs or knock knees, a weak ribcage, and possible deformities in the pelvis.

In adults, vitamin D deficiency manifests as the disease osteomalacia. In this condition, bones lose their mineral content and weaken, increasing the chance of breaks. Pregnant women and the elderly are most susceptible to osteomalacia.

Nutrition Morsels

The diseases osteomalacia and osteoporosis both affect the elderly. Osteomalacia comes from a deficiency of vitamin D, which causes bone demineralization. Demineralization is the progressive loss of calcium and other minerals from bone, which eventually weakens the bone structure and makes bone easier to break.

Osteoporosis is a disease of aging in which bone gradually loses calcium. This also leads to a weakening of bone and the increased risk of breaking. Osteoporosis is not, however, related to vitamin D deficiency.

Vitamin D does not build up in the body as much as vitamin A does, so toxicity is of slightly less concern. Too much vitamin D can, nevertheless, cause too much absorption of calcium by the intestines. The extra calcium starts to lodge in the kidneys and other organs and interferes with their functioning.

Excess calcium in the blood leads to nausea, vomiting, loss of appetite, weakness, and confusion. A person will also experience increased urination as the kidneys struggle to clear the extra calcium from the body.

Excessive exposure to sunlight does not cause vitamin D toxicity because the body stops making new vitamin as soon as it has enough.

Anyone consuming more than 50 micrograms of vitamin D per day for prolonged periods is at risk of developing vitamin D toxicity.

Vitamin E

Vitamin E works inside cell membranes. In the membrane, it exerts strong antioxidant activity. This is particularly important in membranes because they contain large amounts of fatty acids, and fatty acids have a high risk of giving off damaging chemicals called free radicals. Antioxidants of all types are crucial in protecting the body against damage from these highly reactive free radicals.

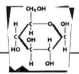

The Chemistry of Nutrition

Free radicals are chemicals that react very readily with other chemicals in the body, especially fats. This high reactivity is due to extra electrons that temporarily cling to the chemical. Free radicals originate in normal cell reactions involving oxygen. Although these reactions may be necessary in normal metabolism, your cells must continually scramble to neutralize the free radicals that form during the body's chemical reactions. Antioxidants take on this vital role. Without antioxidants, free radicals would start a chain reaction of damage to cells, membranes, and enzymes.

Your diet's main antioxidants are vitamin E, vitamin C, and β-carotene. The minerals selenium, zinc, and copper also pitch in some antioxidant activity. A diet with a variety of fresh fruits (especially berries), fresh vegetables, whole grains, and legumes will supply you with the antioxidants you need for good health.

Vitamin E belongs to a family of chemicals called tocopherols. Alpha-, beta-, gamma-, and delta-tocopherol are all forms of the vitamin, with alpha-tocopherol (α-tocopherol) being the most potent form and the main tocopherol in the human body.

Vitamin E Requirements

Nutritionists recommend that adults get 15 milligrams (22 IU) of α-tocopherol daily. Plant oils are the best source:

> ➤ Sunflower oil
> ➤ Safflower oil
> ➤ Canola oil
> ➤ Peanut oil
> ➤ Mayonnaise
> ➤ Salad dressings

Other good sources of vitamin E are:

> ➤ Asparagus
> ➤ Tomatoes
> ➤ Seeds (for example, sunflower seeds)
> ➤ Whole grains
> ➤ Wheat germ
> ➤ Nuts (especially almonds)
> ➤ Peanut butter
> ➤ Some fresh fruits (avocado, papaya, mango, and apples)
> ➤ Some fresh vegetables (kale, broccoli, collard greens, chard, bell peppers, and turnip greens)

Vitamin E Deficiency and Toxicity

Vitamin E deficiency leads to damage of your cell membranes. How do you detect such a microscopic event in the body? A principal symptom shows up as hemolysis, the breakdown of red blood cells. Other symptoms that could occur in E deficiency are muscle weakness, heart muscle damage, and nervous system irregularities.

For a long time, scientists could find little evidence of vitamin E toxicity. For this reason and because of its antioxidant value, people began taking massive amounts of vitamin E daily. Prolonged use of vitamin E supplements of more than 1,000 milligrams per day is now known to interfere with the metabolism of other nutrients. For example, this level of vitamin E intake disrupts the role of vitamin K in normal blood clotting. The symptom for this is abnormal bleeding and bruising.

Vitamin E Supplements

Nutritionists view vitamin E not as a single chemical but rather a group of tocopherols and related compounds called tocotrienols. Pill supplements usually contain a mixture of these chemicals. You will notice these supplements labeled Mixed Tocopherol or "Mixed Tocotrienol."

Many studies have been conducted on vitamin E supplements to determine if they work as well or better than the natural vitamin. The data are still accumulating, but the trends indicate that the supplements do not deliver the same benefits as natural vitamin. Natural vitamin E appears to be better at preventing cardiovascular diseases, affecting the development of prostate cancer, and lowering the risk of respiratory disease. Of course, these diseases result from many factors of dietary, genetic, and lifestyle origins. Although vitamin E has been credited with being a solution to diverse health problems, its role is not easy to pin down. Vitamins interact with other nutrients in body metabolism. Nutritionists cannot evaluate a single nutrient all by itself.

Vitamin K

Vitamin K's main job in the body is as an integral component in blood clotting. Blood must form clots in special instances such as when there are wounds, cuts, burns, and trauma to internal organs. Clotting prevents excessive blood loss. Blood clots also form around infections. The clot keeps pathogens from escaping the immediate area of infection and spreading throughout the body. To carry out its role in clotting, or blood coagulation, vitamin K works in conjunction with specific clotting proteins and calcium. The coagulation process follows several specific steps in order:

1. Tissue damage causes vitamin K to activate clotting factors that circulate in blood in an inactive form. Calcium helps this activation.

2. The activated clotting factors then activate the protein prothrombin.

3. Prothrombin converts into the protein thrombin.

4. Thrombin activates the protein fibrinogen, which is dissolved in blood, and it turns into insoluble fibrin.

5. The threadlike protein fibrin begins building a clot that traps other blood components to seal off an injury or infection.

Without vitamin K, this cascade of events cannot begin. Vitamin K also contributes to the normal development of bone, muscle, and kidneys.

Vitamin K Requirements

Most adults get more than the 90–120 micrograms of vitamin K needed daily. Green, leafy vegetables such as spinach, kale, turnip greens, and dark lettuces provide the best sources. Other good sources are liver and soybean and canola oils. Even some chocolates are fortified with vitamin K.

Vitamin K Deficiency and Toxicity

The prolonged bleeding and bruising associated with vitamin K deficiency is most common in the elderly. Severe deficiency also increases the risk of bone fractures. Vitamin K supplements are often prescribed for the elderly.

No vitamin K toxicities are currently known.

How We Digest Fat-Soluble Vitamins

Fat-soluble vitamins come into our body with dietary fats and are absorbed from the intestines with fats. This is one important reason for having some fat in your diet even when trying to lose weight. Even at our best, we absorb only about 70 percent of dietary fat-soluble vitamins.

Diseases that decrease fat absorption also affect the uptake of fat-soluble vitamins. Cystic fibrosis and Crohn's disease both harm the normal digestion and uptake of fat-soluble vitamins.

Where Fat-Soluble Vitamins Go Inside the Body

After being absorbed, fat-soluble vitamins travel through the bloodstream in the same globules that transport fats, fatty acids, and cholesterol. They are stored mainly in the liver and adipose tissue.

CHAPTER 17

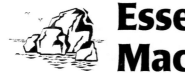 # Essential Minerals: Macrominerals

In This Chapter

➤ The difference between macro- and micro-minerals

➤ Roles, requirements, and sources of macro-minerals

➤ Macro-mineral deficiencies and interactions

In this chapter you will meet the macro-minerals, also called the major minerals. We need these minerals in gram amounts in the diet. The body stores large amounts of these minerals in bone and organs. Micro-minerals, by contrast, are needed in very tiny amounts measured in micrograms or less, and they occur in the body in similarly small amounts.

The macro-minerals covered in this chapter are calcium, magnesium, phosphorus, potassium, and sulfur. Two additional macro-minerals, sodium and chloride, are discussed in the chapter on salt. Macro-minerals play a big part in carbohydrate, fat, protein, and nucleic acid metabolism. Your systems and some organs would quickly shut down without these essential minerals.

What is a Mineral?

A mineral is a chemical element that is not carbon, oxygen, nitrogen, hydrogen, or any other nonmetal. Minerals are therefore always inorganic chemicals from the earth. They usually occur in nature in solid form. If your body were to decompose into its component chemicals, all the minerals would belong to a category called ash. Ash is any noncombustible inorganic material that makes up part of all living and nonliving things on Earth.

We get minerals from both plant and animal foods. Minerals in animal foods tend to be easier to absorb because plant minerals are often bound tightly to plant fibers. Also, plants of the same type can vary greatly in mineral content depending on their soil's mineral supply. As plant foods become more and more processed, their mineral content decreases. For example, wheat grain is a good source of magnesium and micro-minerals, but the mineral content decreases in whole wheat flour. The mineral content declines more when whole wheat flour is refined to white flour:

➤ Whole wheat flour: Calcium, 41 grams; magnesium, 166 milligrams; and selenium, 85 micrograms

➤ White flour: Calcium, 19 grams; magnesium, 27 milligrams; and selenium, 42 micrograms

Minerals serve us by participating in the body's chemical reactions and in forming body structures.

Calcium

Calcium is the mineral that occurs in the largest amounts in the body. You have about 2.5 pounds of calcium inside you, almost all of it in bone and teeth. The skeleton of a growing fetus and a newborn needs a steady supply of calcium, and your calcium demand doesn't stop when you reach adulthood. Calcium works in tandem with phosphorus to maintain healthy bones throughout your life. Outside the skeleton, calcium is essential for blood clotting, transmission of nerve signals, muscle contraction, and the activities of certain enzymes and hormones. It occurs in almost all cells of the body except red blood cells.

An adult absorbs only about 25 percent of dietary calcium, and absorption becomes worse as we age. Absorption is controlled by parathyroid hormone and, fortunately, when the body needs extra calcium, this hormone increases our ability to absorb the mineral. Therefore, pregnant women and growing children are efficient at absorbing calcium.

Calcium Requirements

Adults need from 1 to 1.2 grams of calcium daily. Although calcium is stored in bone, it can escape from bone in a process called demineralization. Dietary calcium must replace the calcium lost in urine and feces.

Calcium Sources

If you eat the recommended servings of dairy products, you get about a third of your calcium needs. Milk and cheese (other than cottage cheese) are excellent sources of calcium.

Other good sources are fortified orange juice, spinach, broccoli, and canned salmon and sardines. Many processed foods are now calcium fortified, so look for this information on the label.

The skeleton acts as a massive calcium storehouse for the rest of the body's cells. For this reason, calcium deficiency in adults is rare.

Magnesium

The body contains a couple of grams of magnesium, distributed about 50:50 between the skeleton and the soft organs. Magnesium is a cofactor in at least three hundred enzymes, many of which function in energy metabolism. You would not be able to get energy from carbohydrates and fats or build protein without magnesium. This mineral is also required for proper cell reproduction, nerve function, and heart activity.

Magnesium Requirements

The body needs 310–400 milligrams of magnesium daily. Men consume and use more magnesium than women. The surface of bone provides a large reserve of magnesium for the rest of the body. Deficiency is unusual and may occur slowly and gradually as magnesium leaches from the skeleton.

Magnesium deficiency causes irregular heartbeats, muscle pain, weakness, and nervous system problems such as seizures.

Magnesium Sources

Several diverse foods supply us with magnesium. Milk, meat, potatoes, vegetables (broccoli, squash, and beans), nuts, seeds, whole grains, and wheat germ are good sources of this mineral.

Phosphorus

Phosphorus works with calcium to keep your bones strong, and bone holds about 85 percent of your body's total phosphorus. Phosphorus is also a critical component of many enzymes, coenzymes, ATP, nucleic acids, and cell membranes. In biology, phosphorus occurs mainly as part of a phosphate group, which is a cluster of phosphorus and oxygen atoms that can attach to other chemicals. Chemists' shorthand for phosphate is PO_4, which stands for one phosphorus (P) connected to four oxygen atoms (O_4).

Phosphate is essential for transporting various nutrients into cells. Some sugars cross membranes only when they have a phosphate group attached to them. In this way, phosphate is vital in all plant, animal, and microbial metabolism.

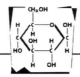

The Chemistry of Nutrition

Phosphorylation is a word only a chemist could love, but it represents an important chemical process that keeps your body running. Phosphorylation is a reaction run by an enzyme that puts a phosphate on a compound. This process is crucial to the body in numerous ways, but the main roles of phosphorylation are to activate energy-yielding reactions involving carbohydrates and fats, activate protein, produce the energy compound ATP, transport sugars across membranes, and work in various mechanisms that control cell metabolism.

Phosphorus Requirements

Adults should consume about 700 milligrams of phosphorus daily. It is likely that we routinely take in much more, but toxicity symptoms do not appear unless a person eats gram amounts of this mineral. A greater worry than phosphorus overdose is imbalance between phosphorus and calcium. These two minerals must be in proper ratios for the best absorption and for maintaining healthy bone.

No phosphorus deficiency diseases have been identified. Any deficiency of phosphorus would likely upset the balance needed between calcium and phosphorus to support normal bone structure and function. Because of phosphorus' importance in bone development, people younger than eighteen years old should consume about 1,250 milligrams daily.

Calcium, Phosphorus, and Bone

Bones depend on the interactions between calcium and phosphorus. The skeleton is not an inert frame upon which you drape your nerves and muscles. Bone is a dynamic structure that takes in calcium and phosphorus and other minerals, such as magnesium, and liberates needed amounts of these minerals to feed metabolism. Bone responds to certain activities that a person might engage in. A mountain climber develops stout long bones of the legs after years of climbing. A construction worker will develop strong bones of the arms and shoulders after years of moving heavy objects.

Bone stores about 99 percent of the body's calcium and 80 percent of its phosphorus. Vitamin D is a major controller of the deposition and removal (demineralization) of these minerals. Both minerals assemble into bone in a specific chemical complex called hydroxyapatite, which contains 10 calcium atoms (Ca) and six phosphates.

Calcium and phosphorus should be absorbed from the gut and enter the bloodstream in about a 2-to-1 ratio. This calcium-phosphorus relationship works best for maintaining healthy bone with the help of vitamin D. Vitamin D not only controls calcium and phosphorus uptake from the gut, but also mediates its deposit and removal in bone. By doing this, the vitamin helps keep your blood calcium and phosphorus ratio at an ideal ratio of about 2.5 to 1.

Different species vary in the optimal calcium-phosphorus ratio they should maintain, and even different people can have slightly different optimal ratios. In general, a ratio of calcium to phosphorus that is too high for several weeks to months will cause extra calcium to be deposited in the body's soft tissues. This causes organ damage. A ratio of too much phosphorus relative to calcium damages bone.

Phosphorus Sources

Good phosphorus sources are:

➤ Dairy products

➤ Meat

➤ Fish

➤ Bread

➤ Eggs

➤ Bran

➤ Breakfast cereals

➤ Sunflower seeds

➤ Nuts (almonds)

You may be surprised, or even pleased, to learn that soft drinks provide a good source of phosphorus from the ingredient phosphoric acid.

Potassium

Potassium is one of several minerals known as electrolytes. It serves to maintain the body's water balance, the amount of water inside cells relative to the outside. Potassium also helps cells balance internal electrical charges with the charges outside the cell. Nerve fibers depend on potassium and inner-outer charge differences to conduct nerve impulses.

Potassium Requirements

Most adults consume up to 3 grams of potassium a day because it is widespread in foods. But nutritionists have determined that we need about 4.7 grams daily. Diets slanted toward fast food and processed foods leave us short in potassium. Fortunately, the body is very good at absorbing almost all the potassium we ingest.

Potassium Deficiency

Low potassium levels in the blood can lead to muscle cramps, constipation, and loss of appetite. Prolonged deficiency causes mental confusion and irregular heartbeat. If the deficiency is prolonged enough to damage the heart muscle, the situation becomes life-threatening because the heart fails to pump adequate blood to the rest of the body.

People who take diuretic drugs for control of high blood pressure or weight loss have a higher risk of becoming potassium deficient because extra mineral gets cleared from the body with increased urine output. Eating disorders, such as bulimia, and alcohol abuse also severely limit a person's capacity to get enough potassium. Even healthy people may be on the borderline for potassium deficiency: people participating in vigorous athletic activity and those on very low-calorie diets run the risk of falling short on potassium.

Potassium Sources

To boost your potassium intake, substitute fresh and unprocessed foods for most of the processed foods you eat. Fruits (especially cantaloupe and banana), vegetables, whole grains, and dried beans deliver fair amounts of potassium. Milk and other dairy products also help.

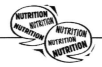

Nutrition Vocabulary

Electrolytes are chemicals that separate into positive and negative versions when dissolved in water. By separating their charges, electrolytes are able to conduct an electrical current. The body's nervous system relies on such electrical conductance to send impulses along nerve fibers. The body's main electrolytes are potassium (K^+), sodium (Na^+), and chloride (Cl^-).

Sulfur

Sulfur is part of the essential amino acids methionine and cysteine—you cannot make protein properly without sulfur—and the vitamins thiamin and biotin. Sulfur also functions in compounds of the liver that detoxify drugs.

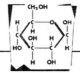

The Chemistry of Nutrition

In nature, sulfur-containing chemicals give off an unpleasant odor due to a portion of the compound called sulfhydryl, or thiol. Sulfhydryl groups are composed simply of sulfur and hydrogen; chemists write it -SH. Sulfhydryl groups vaporize when certain compounds break down in nature. This is what you smell when you detect odors from stagnant swamps, sulfur springs, and hard-boiled eggs! Sulfhydryl is the reason for describing these things as having a rotten egg smell.

Aesthetics aside, sulfhydryls are incredibly important in biology. By connecting to each other during protein formation, they give enzymes and other proteins their necessary structure and activity. Many enzymes cannot work at all without an intact sulfhydryl attached to it. Additionally, the sulfhydryls attached to the protein myosin are needed for normal contraction and relaxation of muscles.

Sulfur Requirements

Protein-rich foods do a good job in fulfilling the body's sulfur needs. Include eggs, meat, dairy products, legumes, and dried beans in your balanced diet. No deficiency symptoms or toxicity problems are associated with dietary sulfur.

How We Digest Minerals

All minerals must dissolve in the watery contents of the intestines to be absorbed. A critical aspect of mineral use relates to bioavailability. Bioavailability is the extent to which a nutrient dissolves and can be absorbed so that the body can use it. As mentioned, a diet high in fiber decreases calcium bioavailability due to a component of vegetables that makes up to 95 percent of the calcium in plant foods unavailable. Oxalic acid and phytic acid are the most important plant constituents that affect calcium bioavailability:

➤ Oxalic acid, or oxalate: Part of many fresh green, leafy vegetables, such as spinach, this compound binds to calcium and further lowers our ability to absorb this mineral.

➤ Phytic acid, or phytate: This compound is a constituent of fiber and also binds to calcium as well as magnesium, iron, zinc, and other essential minerals. Phytic acid is a common constituent in the fibers of grains and beans.

Some animals have an enzyme that breaks apart the phytic acid to release the mineral caught inside it, but humans would do better by eating an omnivorous diet of animal and plant foods. Such a mixture of mineral sources is the best way to increase all minerals' bioavailability.

Mineral Interactions

Oxalic and phytic acids give examples of how minerals interact with specific substances in foods to affect the mineral's digestion. Minerals also interact with vitamins and other minerals in the digestive tract in ways that influence absorption. The following examples show how nutrient-mineral interactions affect absorption:

➤ Vitamin D improves calcium absorption.

➤ Vitamin C improves iron absorption.

➤ Several minerals interfere with each other's uptake, such as the interactions of magnesium, calcium, iron, and copper.

➤ Compounds containing multiple phosphates interfere with the absorption of iron, copper, and zinc.

➤ A calcium-phosphorus ratio between 1 to 1 and 2 to 1 works best for the absorption of both minerals. (Other species require slightly different ratios.)

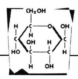

The Chemistry of Nutrition

Electrolytes in the blood and in tissue act in cooperation to maintain the body's acid-base balance. Your body must never become too acidic or too alkaline (basic) because either of these circumstances will shut down enzyme, muscle, and nerve function. A group of electrolytes constantly shuttle into and out of cells for the purpose of keeping acid-base balance on an even keel. Chlorine, phosphorus, and sulfur react with hydrogen to form acid when the body becomes too alkaline. Sodium, magnesium, calcium, and potassium do the opposite; they make conditions more alkaline if conditions are too acidic. Sodium, chloride, and potassium are particularly active in maintaining both the proper acid-base balance and the body's electrolyte balance.

Where Minerals Go Inside the Body

Calcium, phosphorus, and magnesium are stored mainly in bone. But these and other minerals are also dispersed in smaller amounts in every cell of the body. Minerals tend to associate with proteins, such as enzymes, and hormones. The body does not store significant amounts of minerals in fat because minerals tend to dissolve in aqueous solutions in the body. When not bound to a protein, minerals are dissolved in the blood, lymph, interstitial fluid, and the fluid inside individual cells, called cytoplasm.

The kidneys excrete large amounts of minerals every day. This explains why you must eat a variety of mineral-containing foods every day for peak health.

CHAPTER 18

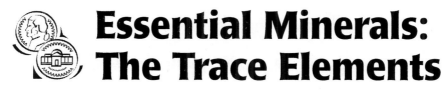

Essential Minerals: The Trace Elements

In This Chapter

➤ Roles, requirements, and sources of trace minerals

➤ Trace mineral deficiencies and potential toxicities

In this chapter you will learn about the minerals needed in the smallest amounts in your diet. These micro-minerals may not take up much space in the body, but they have important roles in enzyme function and the activation of certain vitamins, hormones, and specialized cellular processes.

The micro-minerals are also called trace minerals or trace elements because we need them in the diet and use them in the body in trace amounts. What is a trace amount in a diet consisting of thousands of calories and several grams of food? Trace minerals are needed at levels of 100 milligrams or less each day. Sometimes the requirement reaches only microgram levels. You may also hear the term *parts per million* to describe trace element requirements. This chapter describes how trace elements work in these tiny amounts in the body.

This chapter covers trace elements you probably know your body needs, such as iron and zinc, and others you may not have realized play a key role in health.

Iron

Iron is the part of hemoglobin in red blood cells and myoglobin in muscle that carries oxygen. You therefore need iron to deliver oxygen to cells for respiration. Iron also helps out by carrying away some of the carbon dioxide produced by respiring cells in energy production.

Think of iron in your body the same way you think of gold in a financial sense: it is valuable and not to be treated casually. Iron makes up only 0.004 percent or less of your body; very little iron is stored in the liver, kidneys, and spleen; iron is difficult to absorb; and absorption is strictly controlled because the kidneys do not easily excrete excess iron. Vitamin C is one of the main controllers of iron uptake from the gut. Eating foods rich in vitamin C or drinking orange juice with iron supplements helps iron absorption.

Iron Requirements

Iron deficiency is one of the most common nutrient deficiencies worldwide despite iron's abundance in nature. This metal makes up almost 5 percent of Earth's crust. Your body carries about 5 grams of iron!

Women tend to be more iron deficient than men, so nutritional recommendations focus on women with special recommendations for pregnant or lactating women. Women from around nineteen to fifty years of age have higher iron needs because of losses during menstruation. The current daily recommendations are:

➤ Infants seven to twelve months: 11 milligrams (mg)

➤ Toddlers one to three years: 7 mg

➤ Children four to eight years: 10 mg

➤ Children nine to thirteen years: 8 mg

➤ Young adults fourteen to eighteen years: 15 mg for females, 11 mg for males

➤ Adults nineteen to fifty years: 18 mg for females, 8 mg for males

➤ Older adults: 8 mg

Newborns have a supply of iron from their mother that lasts about six months, so no recommendations have been made for them.

Iron Deficiency

Iron deficiency causes anemia, which is any decreased oxygen-carrying capacity of blood. Physicians might check for possible iron deficiency in patients who are pale, tire easily, or are often short of breath. Two blood tests give an indication of your iron status:

➤ Hematocrit: Percentage of red blood cells in the blood. Normal levels are about 47 percent for men and 42 percent for women.

➤ Hemoglobin concentration: Amount of fully functional hemoglobin in blood. Normal levels are 14–18 grams per 100 milliliters (g/100 ml) blood in men and 12–16 g/100 ml in women.

In addition to blood loss from menstruation or injury or other trauma, deficiency can occur due to certain dietary substances that interfere with absorption. Oxalic acid and phytic acid bind iron and can lead to deficiency.

Iron Sources

Nutritionists divide dietary iron sources into two types: heme and nonheme. Heme is the portion of hemoglobin that clasps onto an iron atom for carrying oxygen. Heme sources of iron are foods that give you fully formed hemoglobin. In other words, these are animal food sources. Nonheme sources of iron force you to make your own hemoglobin from dietary iron.

The top sources of heme iron are:

➤ Chicken or beef liver

➤ Oysters

➤ Beef (steaks and roasts)

➤ Shrimp

➤ Tuna

➤ Halibut

➤ Poultry

➤ Crab

The best sources of nonheme iron are:

➤ Iron-fortified cereals and oatmeal

➤ Soybeans (including tofu) and other beans (kidney, navy, lima, black, and pinto)

➤ Lentils

➤ Black-eyed peas

➤ Molasses (blackstrap)

➤ Spinach

Milk and milk products are poor sources of iron.

Nutrition Vocabulary

Some nutrients are present in foods in amounts so small that scientists could not accurately measure them until they invented more sensitive instruments. Some trace elements are measured in units called parts per million, or ppm. A ppm is one part of a substance in a million equal parts of something else. For example, a drop of oil in a 15-gallon trash can filled with water is 1 ppm.

Some trace elements and harmful chemicals might show up in your food at levels even lower than ppm. Chemists now measure things to the level of parts per billion (ppb) and parts per trillion (ppt) and will soon be able to get accurate measurements of ever smaller quantities of chemicals. An example of a ppb is one sunflower seed in a 45-foot silo filled with corn kernels. One ppt is 1 square foot of land in the entire state of Indiana.

Zinc

We absorb less than 50 percent of dietary zinc, and zinc deficiency is not uncommon in even well-fed parts of the world. This mineral makes up 0.02 percent of Earth's crust.

The human body holds only about 3 milligrams of zinc, but this mineral shows up in at least two hundred different enzymes. These enzymes work in diverse systems:

➤ DNA function

➤ Protein metabolism

➤ Cell membrane integrity

➤ Wound healing

➤ Immunity

➤ Development of reproductive organs

Zinc also acts as an antioxidant. Most of your zinc stays in skin and hair. Very small amounts occur in bone, muscles, organs, and blood.

Zinc may participate in eye health and vision because megadoses (80 milligrams) have been shown to reduce the development of macular degeneration.

Zinc Requirements

Men require about 11 milligrams of zinc daily, and women should consume 8 milligrams. Most people in North America consume these levels of zinc and perhaps not much more. Nutritionists warn that some groups are likely to be zinc deficient for some part of their life. These groups are women, children in poor families, people who eat no animal foods or foods derived from animals (vegan diet), the elderly, and alcoholics.

Zinc Deficiency

Symptoms of zinc deficiency are:

➤ Growth retardation

➤ Poor development of sexual organs and the skeleton

➤ Skin rashes

➤ Diarrhea

➤ Loss of appetite

➤ Hair loss

➤ Increased rate of infections

Deficiencies worldwide arise from malnutrition, especially in the young and in people eating a high-fiber diet high in phytic acid.

Zinc Sources

Protein-rich diets usually supply good amounts of zinc. As a person's diet shifts away from animal protein to plant protein, the chance of zinc deficiency rises. Despite the presence of phytic acid, which makes some zinc unavailable to you, whole grains, peanuts, and legumes are good sources. Other good sources of zinc are beef, lamb, pork, chicken, fish (especially cod), fortified cereals, and wheat germ. Perhaps the world championship in supplying zinc goes to raw or steamed oysters, which provide 90 to more than 200 milligrams per about three oysters.

Zinc supplements supply zinc in the form of zinc oxide. These supplements have proven useful in correcting deficiencies and alleviating some of the effects of macular degeneration.

Zinc and copper are known to interfere with each other's bioavailability. Therefore, zinc supplementation should not be a long-term approach to nutrition but rather a temporary action taken under the direction of a doctor or nutritionist.

Nutrition Morsels

Zinc is a key component of many of the enzymes involved in energy generation. For this reason, nutritionists categorize foods based on a quality called zinc energy density. Foods of high zinc energy density provide the body with a good energy source plus enough zinc to run energy-generating reactions after digesting the food. High zinc energy density foods are lamb, leafy vegetables, root vegetables, shellfish, and beef organ meats. Moderate zinc energy density foods are whole grains, pork, poultry, milk, eggs, nuts, and fish. Poor zinc energy density foods are oils, butter, and sugary foods.

Iodine

Iodine works in the body in its ion or charged form called iodide. (The chemical symbol for iodine is *I* and the symbol for iodide is *I⁻*.) Iodide functions in maintaining normal activity of the thyroid gland. A thyroid gland supplied with sufficient iodide then makes thyroid hormones that control growth, development, and metabolic rate.

Iodine Requirements and Sources

Adults need about 150 micrograms of iodide daily. Most of us get this amount in iodized salt; a half teaspoon provides the entire daily requirement. Because most processed foods and fast foods have high amounts of salt, it is likely that many of us consume iodide far in excess of our needs.

If you eat a diet that limits your salt intake, good natural iodide sources are yogurt, buttermilk, low-fat milk, eggs, and cottage cheese.

Iodine Deficiency

An enlarged thyroid gland hints at iodide deficiency. The enlargement is due to the thyroid struggling to take up more iodide from the bloodstream. Such a prolonged stress on the thyroid leads to goiter, a permanent enlargement of this gland.

Nutrition Morsels

Goiter has been known to exist in broad swaths of continents due to a deficiency of iodine in the soils used for growing crops. This type of goiter associated with a geographic region is called endemic goiter and is unrelated to cases of illness that have genetic causes. In the early 1900s, physicians discovered that an endemic goiter belt stretched across the northern United States and into southern Canada.

Today we have eliminated the risk of goiter by using iodized salt. This tactic was first investigated by physician David Marine in Akron in 1916 to successfully prevent goiter in schoolchildren. In later years, the World Health Organization commissioned Marine to institute similar programs for distributing iodized salt. After hearing of Marine's single experiment in Ohio, Michigan physician David Cowie encouraged salt manufacturers to routinely iodize salt for preventing goiter in the larger U.S. population.

Salt manufacturers now spray potassium iodide (KI) onto crystals of table salt to make iodized salt. Pure table salt is sodium chloride (NaCl). Iodized table salt is sodium chloride plus about 0.004 percent potassium iodide.

Copper

Copper is widespread in the Earth's crust and is fairly well absorbed by the digestive tract. Adults can absorb up to 75 percent of dietary copper. Other substances in the diet can, however, interfere with absorption:

- ➤ Zinc
- ➤ Iron
- ➤ Molybdenum
- ➤ Vitamin C
- ➤ Some sugars
- ➤ Fibers high in phytic acid

The body uses copper as enzyme cofactors. A wide variety of enzymes require copper for activity. Some of the main copper enzyme activities are:

- ➤ Electron transport chain reactions in respiration and ATP production
- ➤ Control of some brain neurotransmitters
- ➤ Steps in hemoglobin synthesis and blood clotting
- ➤ Melanin synthesis
- ➤ Synthesis of the proteins elastin and collagen
- ➤ Contributes to iron metabolism

Copper Requirements and Sources

Adults need about 900 micrograms of copper daily and most people probably get adequate amounts from a balanced diet. Dietary sources are thought to be much more available to the body than supplements.

The best dietary sources of copper are:

- ➤ Beef liver
- ➤ Seafood (especially lobster and shrimp)
- ➤ Legumes
- ➤ Whole grain breads and cereals
- ➤ Molasses
- ➤ Nuts

> ➤ Cocoa
> ➤ Sunflower seeds

Copper Deficiency

Copper deficiency symptoms are anemia, low white blood cell count, poor growth in the young, and bone loss.

Selenium

Selenium deficiencies and toxicities have been found in specific geographic regions worldwide. Selenium is easily absorbed. Because selenium is chemically similar to sulfur, it can substitute for sulfur in amino acids such as cysteine (selenocysteine) and methionine (selenomethionine). Proteins that have selenium instead of sulfur can usually function normally. About thirty proteins in the body are known to replace selenium for sulfur in cysteine and methionine without any health risks.

Selenium's main function is as an antioxidant. Vitamin E and selenium often work together to protect cells against peroxides formed during oxygen reactions. When working together, the vitamin tends to protect the cell membrane and selenium protects the aqueous parts of the cell. Selenium performs its antioxidant role by being part of the enzyme glutathione peroxidase. This enzyme neutralizes the harmful effects of hydrogen peroxide and the peroxides that form during lipid metabolism.

Selenium Requirements and Sources

Adults should consume 55 micrograms of selenium daily. Most people take in more than this amount. Soils in the Pacific Northwest, the Great Lakes states, the mid-Atlantic region, and New England can be deficient in selenium. This might have been a nutritional problem last century when people grew their own crops. Today's global distribution of foods makes selenium deficiency an almost nonexistent problem.

The best sources for selenium are:

> ➤ Fish and shellfish
> ➤ Organ meats
> ➤ Eggs
> ➤ Grains and seeds grown in selenium-rich soils

Selenium Deficiency and Toxicity

Selenium deficiency's main symptoms are muscle pain and wasting disease, which is a heart disorder caused by a decline in heart muscle function and a breakdown of muscle fats. These symptoms develop because of decreased activity of glutathione peroxidase. In severely deficient parts of the world (northern China and eastern Siberia), people may develop Kashin-Beck disease characterized by a weakening of joint cartilage.

Because localized regions of the world have very high soil selenium levels, toxicity may be more of a concern than deficiency. Soils in parts of the Plains states contain high selenium concentrations. People who consume grains or seeds grown in these soils or who take more than 400 micrograms of selenium daily will experience selenium toxicity symptoms: hair loss, nail brittleness and loss, skin rashes, intestinal disturbances, and various nervous system abnormalities.

Manganese

Manganese is often confused for magnesium because their names are similar and because these two minerals often substitute for each other in enzymes. Manganese also has specific roles in carbohydrate metabolism, control of free radicals, and bone formation.

People need only 1.8–2.3 milligrams of manganese a day and likely get this amount from a balanced diet. Whole grains, nuts, beans, and leafy vegetables are good sources.

Fluorine

Fluorine is like iodine because the body uses it in a charged form called fluoride (F^-). (Fluorine, iodine, and chlorine all belong to the same chemical group of elements and behave similarly in chemical reactions.)

Nutritionists consider fluoride to be a nutrient based on its value in bone and tooth enamel development in children. Fluoride combines with calcium and enters rebuilding bone in the form of a crystal compound called calcium fluorapatite. Dentists recommend that fluoride-containing toothpastes be used by people of all ages to replace bone loss from enamel and protect against dental caries. Many communities also put fluoride into municipal drinking water to help people get their fluoride. Bottled water lacks fluoride.

Other than its role in bone health, the functions of fluoride in the body are poorly understood. It is known to activate some enzymes and deactivate others.

Some nutritionists debate whether fluoride is an essential nutrient despite its benefits in bone and tooth health. Nutrition resources often disagree on whether people need to consume small amounts of fluoride or merely apply it regularly to teeth with toothpaste.

If a person does not use fluoridated toothpastes or drink fluoridated water, they should consider adding a food source of fluoride to the diet. Tea, seafood, and seaweed are sources of dietary fluoride.

Nutrition Morsels

Water fluoridation is the process of adding fluoride to municipal drinking water. Since cities began adding 1 ppm fluoride to water in the 1940s the incidence of dental caries in North America has steadily declined. Most health professionals, public water utilities, and the U.S. Department of Health and Human Services support the use of fluoridated water as a benefit to community health.

Fluoridated water is not universally accepted, however. Some communities have resisted water fluoridation because of fears of fluoride toxicity. Health professionals and researchers have weighed in with their concerns about the potential hazards of adding small but constant doses of fluoride to everyone's diet. Fluorosis is chronic fluoride poisoning evident as mottling of the tooth enamel, particularly in children. Although fluorosis is known to arise from high exposures to fluoride, water fluoridation has never been proven to be its cause.

The U.S. Department of Health and Human Services has recently adjusted the recommended fluoridation level to 0.7 ppm, although it continues to promote fluoridation for health and investigate any potential hazards from fluoride.

Chromium

Chromium is one of nutrition's most recent additions to our list of essential nutrients. This metal is known to be toxic in high doses yet is needed in small doses for proper insulin function. Chromium helps the hormone transport glucose into cells.

Whole grains, meat, and foods from yeast, including beer, are good sources. The chromium requirement is about 30 micrograms per day.

Chromium toxicity occurs in places where industrial pollution has tainted groundwater, surface waters, and soil. Liver damage and lung cancer are known consequences of chromium toxicity. This metal accumulates in those organs as well as in the heart, spleen, and muscle.

Molybdenum

Molybdenum is another metal used in spare amounts in select enzymes. The body easily absorbs molybdenum and it is found in all tissues. It functions in the enzymes of respiration that also require iron and riboflavin. Molybdenum enzymes also play a role in certain catabolic reactions, such as the breakdown of nucleic acids to uric acid.

Molybdenum deficiency is rare. Most people can get their required 45 micrograms from beans, nuts, and grains.

The Chemistry of Nutrition

Heavy metals belong to a group of elements (metals) that conduct electrical current, shine, and are made of atoms with a positive charge. Although this group is loosely defined, most chemists would classify the following as heavy metals:

➤ Cadmium

➤ Chromium

➤ Copper

➤ Lead

➤ Mercury

➤ Thallium

➤ Zinc

Some chemists also include:

➤ Iron

➤ Manganese

➤ Molybdenum

➤ Cobalt

Some of these have already been mentioned in this book as essential nutrients, while others such as mercury and cadmium are known more for their toxic properties.

The heavy metals may help metabolism at very low concentrations, but high doses (about 2 milligrams daily) cause irreversible damage to the heart, lungs, liver, kidneys, and nervous system. Heavy metal toxicity has emerged as a serious health problem worldwide where soil and/or water is contaminated with industrial pollutants. The toxicities increase as the metal moves up a food chain from plants to animals to other animals that prey on them. Humans, who are at the top of their food chain, can suffer health problems by eating meat or fish contaminated with these metals. The increasing concentration of pollutants moving up a food chain is called bioaccumulation.

Other Elements We May Need in Tiny Amounts

Nutritionists have identified other trace elements that may have jobs in body metabolism. Because these nutrients are needed in miniscule amounts, we can easily meet our daily needs for them, so few deficiency symptoms are known.

Thirteen elements have been proposed as potential trace elements, but we need to learn more about how they work in the body and if they are truly required:

1. Aluminum

2. Arsenic

3. Boron

4. Bromine

5. Cadmium

6. Germanium

7. Lead

8. Lithium

9. Nickel

10. Rubidium

11. Silicon

12. Tin

13. Vanadium

Chromium used to belong to this group until its role in glucose uptake by cells was confirmed.

Mineral Toxicity

Sometimes nutritionists know more about a trace element's toxicity in the human body than its role as a nutrient. We need trace elements in such tiny amounts that it can be easier to get too much than too little. This is particularly true for people who take supplements without professional supervision.

In the body most trace elements bind to protein. Sometimes, perhaps most of the time, this association causes no harm. If a trace element interferes, however, with the normal structure and reactive regions on a protein, an important process in metabolism can be affected.

A single enzyme, which you have likely never heard of, can falter under the influence of high amounts of a trace element. In turn, metabolism does not run at its best. In the worst circumstances, trace element toxicity leads to cancers, liver damage, kidney damage, and other organ malfunctions.

Beware of the following upper limits for safely consuming minerals:

- ➤ Chloride: 3.6 grams
- ➤ Sodium: 2.3 grams
- ➤ Calcium: 2.5 grams
- ➤ Phosphorus: 3–4 grams
- ➤ Magnesium: 350 milligrams
- ➤ Iron: 45 milligrams
- ➤ Zinc: 40 milligrams
- ➤ Manganese: 11 milligrams
- ➤ Copper: 10 milligrams
- ➤ Fluoride: 10 milligrams
- ➤ Molybdenum: 2 milligrams
- ➤ Iodide: 1.1 milligrams
- ➤ Selenium: 400 micrograms

CHAPTER 19

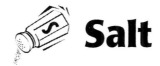 **Salt**

In This Chapter

➤ Characteristics of salt

➤ How the body uses sodium and chloride

➤ Types of salts in biology and in the diet

In this chapter I give special attention to a component of the diet that has a tremendous impact on nutrition and health. It is salt.

Salt is a simple molecule. Chemists write it NaCl, where *Na* stands for sodium and *Cl* refers to chlorine. The *Na* comes from the Latin word *natrium* for sodium. Salt is an important food that supplies these two essential nutrients.

Like sugar, salt has been saddled with a bad reputation in nutrition. Your doctor is as likely to tell you to cut back on your salt intake as much as you are supposed to lower your sugar intake. Yet like sugar, salt is essential in metabolism. You cannot last a day without it. Let's investigate the good things salt does for you.

What Is Salt?

To chemists, plenty of chemicals in addition to NaCl qualify as salts. Any compound made of a positively charged atom combined with a negatively charged atom is a salt. Therefore, potassium chloride (KCl) is as much a salt as sodium chloride is. Chemists also define a salt as any compound resulting from the combination of an acid and a base. For example, sulfuric acid (H_2SO_4) and the base sodium hydroxide (NaOH) can combine to form the salt sodium sulfate (Na_2SO_4). Salt names usually end in *-ate*, *-ite*, or *-ide*.

Types of Salts in Chemistry

By following the rules of combining positive and negative chemicals or acids and bases, you could mix up an almost limitless variety of salts in a laboratory. The following are the major salts that have important roles in biology. They are produced when a negatively charged molecule combines with the positively charged form of calcium (Ca^+), magnesium (Mg^{2+}), potassium (K^+), or sodium (Na^+):

➤ Chlorides: Combine chloride (Cl^-) with a positive molecule

➤ Carbonates: Combine carbonate (CO_3^{2-}) with positive molecules with a charge of +2

➤ Bicarbonates: Combine bicarbonate (HCO_3^-) with a positive molecule

➤ Sulfates: Combine sulfate (SO_4^{2-}) with positive molecules with a total charge of +2

➤ Phosphates: Combine phosphate (PO_4^{3-}) with positive molecules with a total charge of +3

What Salts Do in the Body

Salts have various roles in the bloodstream and tissue when they break apart into their constituent electrolytes. They help maintain osmotic pressure of cells, meaning they help balance pressures on the inside of cells with pressures on the cell's outside. Salts similarly maintain water balance and the body's acid-base balance. They do these things by affecting the permeability of cell membranes.

Salts help the body regulate blood volume; salt levels tell the kidneys whether the blood is too concentrated (low volume) or too dilute (high volume). The kidneys then adjust water output to bring the blood volume back into normal range.

Various salts also have specific jobs in bone and tooth structure, the signal system of nerve and muscle, certain enzymes and hormones, respiratory pigments, and in the steps required for blood clotting.

Sodium

Sodium is a macro-mineral abundant on Earth. It is the sixth most abundant element in Earth's crust and comprises 80 percent of seawater. An adult needs about 1.5 grams of sodium a day, a level that should be reduced to about 150 milligrams as we age. About 80 percent of the sodium we consume comes with the salt added to foods made by food companies or prepared in restaurants. The rest comes in less processed foods. Interestingly, only humans confront the problem of too much salt in highly processed diets. Wildlife and livestock diets are usually deficient in salt.

It's not hard to identify the salty foods in your diet, which supply both sodium and chloride: they taste salty! One of these foods, saltine crackers, tells you one of the main ingredients right in its name. Other sources of sodium are ham, pizza, canned soup, vegetable juice, cheese, and canned vegetables. Frozen prepared meals are a veritable sodium and chloride goldmine.

Most people even on low-salt diets get more than their requirements for sodium and chloride. Only if a high level of perspiration leads to weight loss, such as experienced by endurance athletes and soldiers in training, should sodium deficiency be a concern. Eating salty food is the easiest way to correct the deficiency.

Sodium Deficiency

Sodium deficiency is rare and usually temporary because it is associated with intense physical activity. The symptoms are muscle cramps, dizziness, nausea, and vomiting. Severe, prolonged sodium loss can cause shock, coma, and may lead to death.

Sodium's Role in the Body

The symptoms of sodium deficiency hint at the role this mineral plays in the body. In addition to helping balance osmotic pressure, water, and electrolytes in blood and tissue, sodium plays a central role in these functions:

➤ Nerve signal conduction

➤ Muscle contraction

➤ Transport of nutrients into cells

Nutrition Morsels

The kidneys eliminate excess sodium and chloride, so salt toxicity is not a common concern. But too much dietary salt cannot be dismissed in overall health. Elevated salt in the body leads to hypertension, or high blood pressure. Hypertension occurs when a person's blood pressure consistently stays above 140 millimeters mercury systolic or 90 millimeters mercury diastolic. You might hear the blood pressure reading abbreviated to 140 over 90.

The first number represents the pressure in the arteries when the heart is contracting. This action is called systole. The bottom number refers to the pressure in arteries when the heart is relaxing. This phase of the regular heartbeat is called diastole. Physicians put a little more meaning on the diastolic pressure because of its association with heart attack and stroke.

Blood pressure tends to rise with age, so sodium and chloride levels should be reduced accordingly as you get older. The best way to do this is to eliminate processed foods known to be high in salt.

Chlorine

Our bodies use chlorine in its charged form. This is the ion called chloride (Cl⁻). Chloride comes as a package deal with sodium every time you consume table salt, so chloride deficiency is rare in North America. Some fruits and vegetables are good natural sources of chloride.

Chloride is critical to acid-base balance of body fluids and makes up the acid secreted by the stomach. The stomach's hydrochloric acid (HCl) is important in the breakdown of food particles during digestion. The hydrochloric acid also converts the stomach enzyme pepsinogen to its active form pepsin soon after you have begun eating a meal. Pepsin then starts breaking down the meal's proteins. Chloride is also needed for proper nerve function.

Most people get an excess of chloride in their diet. Deficiencies can occur in the severely malnourished or in people with eating disorders that involve induced vomiting. The vomiting contributes to chloride deficiency because of the loss of gastric juices containing hydrochloric acid.

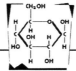

The Chemistry of Nutrition

Chemically, table salt is NaCl. The sodium and chloride are not evenly matched in table salt, however. By the weight of their molecules, table salt is 40 percent sodium and 60 percent chloride. In other words, a teaspoon of salt weighing about 2 grams contains 800 milligrams (0.8 gram) of sodium and 1,200 milligrams (1.2 grams) of chloride.

Types of Salt Important in Nutrition

The term *salt* might not always refer to sodium chloride. Let's distinguish among the many different types of salts that play a role in nutrition. The following are used in foods, some nonfoods, or become active only inside the body:

➤ Bile salts: Salts excreted by the gallbladder to help in the digestion of dietary fat. The main bile salts in humans are sodium taurocholate and sodium glycocholate. The liver makes both bile salts from cholesterol.

➤ Buffer salts: Added to some beverages and candies to keep the food from becoming too acidic or too basic. Examples are potassium citrate and sodium citrate.

➤ Epsom salt: This is magnesium sulfate ($MgSO_4$). It is used to add magnesium to vegetable gardens.

➤ Glauber's salt: This is sodium sulfate (Na_2SO_4). It is sometimes used as a laxative when taken internally.

➤ Iodized salt: This is sodium chloride with a small amount of potassium iodide added to boost your iodide intake.

➤ Neutral salt: Any salt that is neither acidic nor basic; sodium chloride is our most familiar example.

➤ Rock salt: This is the natural form of sodium chloride. Rock salt occurs in dry lakebeds and evaporating marine waters. Its crystals are very coarse and grayish in color. Celtic salt is a form of rock salt harvested from evaporating marsh water.

➤ Sea salt (also bay salt): This is sodium chloride harvested from seawater.

➤ Substitute salts: These are any chemicals that have a salty taste but do not contain sodium. Potassium chloride is the most commonly used salt substitute for people trying to lower their salt (NaCl) intake. Some dried herb blends also tout themselves as substitute salts.

➤ Table salt: Either iodized or non-iodized forms of sodium chloride qualify as table salt.

Types of Salt for Cooking

Table salt has branched out into the gourmet and exotic varieties. All of the salts listed below are derivations of sodium chloride and behave the same way in the body:

➤ Coarse salt: Large crystals like that on pretzels

➤ Kosher salt: Also has a coarser grind than regular table salt, this salt has no additives and adheres to kosher dietary rules

➤ Seasoned salt: Contains various herbs

➤ Colored salts: May be either natural or containing food additives to give the crystals a pink, yellow, orange, reddish, or black color

Salt producers also offer salts in a wide variety of coarseness from very large, irregular crystals to extremely fine powder. These different varieties affect cooking more than they affect nutrition.

Sodium-Containing Food Additives

The food industry has developed a long list of sodium compounds that help with the manufacturing of foods and the enhancement of certain food qualities. Sodium salts are hardly a new idea in food preparation: ancient societies began using salt as a food preservative before the earliest recorded history. In fact, sodium chloride still works very well to preserve foods.

Curing meats is the act of soaking the meat in a brine solution (also called salting) or rubbing a coat of salt over the meat before storing it. This ancient method of preservation keeps microbes from destroying the meat even when it is stored near room temperature, while also enhancing the meat's flavor and texture.

Today's sodium salts used as food additives are:

> ➤ Sodium alginate: Thickener
> ➤ Sodium bicarbonate: Yeast substitute
> ➤ Sodium citrate: Flavor enhancer and preservative
> ➤ Sodium cyclamate: Artificial sweetener
> ➤ Sodium nitrate and sodium nitrite: Preservatives and color fixatives
> ➤ Sodium benzoate and sodium propionate: Preservatives
> ➤ Sodium tripoliphosphate: Binder
> ➤ Sodium aluminosilicate: Anticaking additive
> ➤ Sodium aluminum phosphate and sodium caseinate: Emulsifiers
> ➤ Monosodium glutamate (MSG): Flavor enhancer

The above salts do not have nutritional value other than putting a little more sodium into your diet.

PART FIVE

Total Body Nutrition

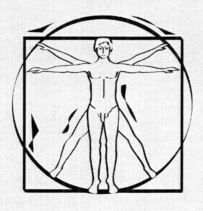

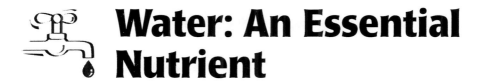

CHAPTER 20

Water: An Essential Nutrient

In This Chapter

➤ The uses of water in the body

➤ How water moves through the body

➤ Best ways to replace water

In this chapter you consider all the benefits of water and learn how water fits into nutrition.

Water is an easily overlooked nutrient. Most nutrition textbooks do not even mention water in their list of essential nutrients. This seems foolish considering nutrients would not be digested, absorbed, transported, or used in metabolism without water. Your body could not eliminate the wastes from metabolism without water. The circulatory system would slow to a trickle then stop without . . . You get the idea.

Let's learn about my favorite nutrient.

Water and Biology

Water is called the universal solvent in biology. This means that almost all biological reactions take place in water. Most nutrients other than lipids and fat-soluble vitamins dissolve in water.

Biological cells contain from 70 to 95 percent water. The adult human male is about 65 percent water and females are around 55 percent water. Newborns contain a higher percentage of water. This simple chemical (H_2O) is present both inside cells and outside cells as it bathes body tissues and organs. The chemical reactions of anabolism and catabolism require water as the material in which they operate.

I could write a second book on the role of water in biology, but let's focus on a general list of how water serves living organisms:

> ➤ The medium in which biochemical reactions occur

> ➤ A chemical involved in certain catabolic reactions called hydrolytic reactions

> ➤ The main transporting agent for substances in the body

> ➤ The main component of the body fluids blood, lymph, cerebral spinal fluid, tissue fluids, saliva, gastric juice, bile, sweat, urine, and intestinal contents

> ➤ The main constituent of intracellular fluid called cytoplasm

> ➤ A solvent for acids, bases, and salts as well as for sugars, amino acids, and other organic compounds

> ➤ A vehicle for transporting red blood cells, which carry oxygen to tissues

> ➤ The substance most important in maintaining constant body temperature

> ➤ A lubricant for organs, nerves, muscle, and joints

> ➤ A cushion surrounding the brain

> ➤ Main vehicle for eliminating wastes and excess vitamins and minerals from the body

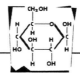

The Chemistry of Nutrition

Hydrolysis is a type of chemical reaction that requires water. From the terms *hydro* for water and *lysis* for splitting, you can assume that a hydrolysis reaction involves the splitting of a water molecule. The body uses hydrolysis when it digests polymers, such as polysaccharides and proteins, in the digestive tract. Hydrolysis is again used when you need to break down glycogen for energy or proteins to release amino acids.

In hydrolysis, a water molecule (H_2O) splits into hydrogen (H) and hydroxyl (OH). Each of these two chemicals then hook onto fragments of the polymer being broken into pieces by an enzyme. For example, a polymer being degraded through hydrolysis would follow this general equation:

—Subunit—Subunit —Subunit—Subunit + H2O →

—Subunit—Subunit—H + HO—Subunit—Subunit -

The enzymes that carry out hydrolysis in the body belong to a broad group called hydrolytic enzymes. They have the general name *hydrolases*. Amylase, sucrase, protease, and lipase are examples of hydrolases.

Your Body's Water

Water moves freely across membranes into and out of cells. This keeps all your cells constantly hydrated. Cells are about 70 percent water by weight and about 99 percent of all the molecules making up your cells are water molecules.

Water moves across cell membranes using the process called osmosis. In osmosis, water crosses a semipermeable membrane in the direction of higher concentration of dissolved materials. (Semipermeable membranes let some substances cross them but halt the flow of other substances.) In other words, if your cells are slightly dehydrated, the concentration of salts and other molecules rises a bit inside the cell. In this situation, water flows into the cell to readjust the concentration of dissolved substances. Conversely, if your cells contain too much water, this water dilutes the cell contents too much. A little water then oozes out of the cell to keep things in balance.

The water inside cells is called intracellular fluid and is the site of many of the enzymatic reactions that run your metabolism. The water outside cells is called extracellular fluid. This is the fluid that makes up blood, lymph, and the water that surrounds organs and the spinal column.

The body stores water in two forms: free and bound. Free water is the liquid form that dissolves things and is available for chemical reactions. Bound water is intracellular water attached to compounds and not available for metabolism. Chemists use a term called *water potential* to predict the direction water will flow based on the concentration of substances on either side of a semipermeable membrane. The whole point of all this flowing into and out of cells is to maintain the body's water balance.

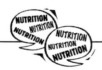

Nutrition Vocabulary

Water balance is a condition in which the body takes in the proper amount of water so that intracellular and extracellular levels are sufficient for your metabolism. Your body alerts you when you are out of water balance by making you feel thirsty or giving you a salt craving. Thirst tells you your body needs more water. Salt cravings indicate that your body has too much water and the substances dissolved in intracellular and extracellular fluids are too diluted.

Water balance is maintained by drinking to take in more water and by sweating and urination to excrete excess water.

Water Elimination

The body eliminates excess water by four routes: perspiration, urination, defecation, and breathing.

Water loss via perspiration ranges from negligible amounts to significant losses. The factors that affect perspiration are:

➤ Environmental temperature

➤ Humidity

➤ Level of physical exertion

➤ Behavioral factors such as nervousness

A person working outdoors on a hot summer day can lose more than 5 quarts of sweat in a few hours.

We should always take in more water than we need because the kidneys need the excess water to eliminate wastes through urination. The wastes produced in normal metabolism get eliminated in urine. Urine always carries away excess water-soluble vitamins, minerals, and drugs. Adults normally produce between 1 and 2 quarts of urine daily, but this can vary quite a bit depending on your age and general health.

Unabsorbed water from beverages and foods are eliminated in the feces. The large intestine reabsorbs most of this dietary water and thus helps maintain your total body water balance. The small volume of extra unabsorbed water helps soften stools for easier defecation.

Only in cases of diarrhea does most of your water loss occur by way of defecation. Diarrhea can be caused by infection, chronic disease, drugs, or certain foods. In diarrhea, too much water passes through the intestines too fast for the body to absorb it all. Severe diarrhea can cause dehydration and even a temporary deficiency of nutrients. Infant diarrhea in many parts of the world is the main factor in malnutrition. This problem is most often caused by infection.

Respiration and the lungs eliminate some water in the form of vapor and very tiny moisture droplets called aerosols.

A healthy adult will eliminate excess water daily by the four main excretion routes in the following approximate proportions:

1. Urine: 6.75 cups

2. Perspiration: 3 cups

3. Lung respiration: 1.25 cups

4. Feces: 0.4 cup

Thirst

The body's thirst mechanism is controlled by the hypothalamus. This structure is attached to the underside of the brain and also helps regulate the nervous system, body temperature, and the pituitary gland.

The body monitors water balance by keeping tabs on blood volume and salt concentration in blood. If water levels are low, the hypothalamus sends a message to the kidneys to conserve water by reabsorbing more during the normal process of filtering blood and making urine. The hypothalamus simultaneously initiates a thirst sensation. This triggers your impulse to drink water, seek a soda machine, or head for the nearest beer vendor at the ballpark!

A dry mouth can activate the thirst mechanism, but certain drugs, foods, and even nervousness can also do this.

Nutrition Morsels

Many places worldwide, including parts of the United States, experience water stress. Water stress occurs when the land in a geographic region cannot meet the water demands of its people, animals, and crops.

Good irrigation systems alleviate water stress in many places, but in developing countries water stress is often a population's greatest health threat. Not only does limited water supply lead to dehydration of the people, it stunts the growth of livestock and crops. The scarce water sources in many parts of the world often contain contamination from chemicals or human and animal wastes. People's risk of disease and infection increases when they are forced to use this contaminated source for drinking and cooking. The World Health Organization cites water stress as one of the world's greatest current health concerns.

Dietary Water

A person should consume about 2.8 quarts of water daily. That's a little more than 11 cups. In general, women need about 9 cups and men should consume about 13 cups. This water can come from tap or bottled water, other beverages, and foods. Many foods, in fact, supply water better than they supply most other nutrients. The following foods contain at least 70 percent water by weight:

➤ Lettuce

➤ Tomatoes

➤ Oranges

➤ Apples

➤ Potatoes

➤ Bananas

If you do not enjoy drinking water, you can also meet your fluid intake requirements with milk, tea, coffee, soft drinks (soda), and juices. Be aware, however, that teas, coffees, and soft drinks can also contain caffeine. Caffeine is a diuretic substance, meaning it increases urine output. If you are trying to hydrate your body with these beverages, seek the decaffeinated versions.

In most diets, most of your water (about 8 cups) comes with drinking water and beverages. You get an additional 2 cups in food and the body's metabolism produces another 1.25 cups from chemical reactions.

Recommended Beverages for Meeting Water Needs

Only water hydrates you without giving you extra calories or any other chemical that your body must process and then eliminate. Drinking plain water is the best way to supply the bulk of your water needs. Nutritionists recommend that other beverages be consumed in lesser amounts according to the following guidelines for a typical North American diet:

➤ Water: 50 fluid ounces, or 6.25 cups

➤ Tea or coffee, unsweetened: 0–40 fluid ounces, or 5 cups

➤ Low-fat, skim milk, or soy beverages: 0–16 fluid ounces, or 2 cups

➤ Diet drinks with no calories: 0–32 fluid ounces, or 4 cups

➤ Juices, sports drinks, whole milk, or alcohol: 0–8 fluid ounces, or 1 cup

➤ Regular soft drinks: 0–8 fluid ounces, or 1 cup

Few nutritionists would encourage you to increase your alcohol or soft drink consumption to fit these guidelines if you don't already drink these beverages.

The above guidelines were published by clinical nutritionist Barry Popkin in 2006. They represent a healthy yet realistic variety of beverages. Unfortunately, most North Americans today do not consume beverages in these proportions or total volumes. The authors of Popkin's study discovered that our drinking habits are more like the list below. Notice the kcal distribution people in the United States are now getting from these beverages:

➤ Water: 50 fluid ounces (0 kcal)

➤ Tea or coffee, unsweetened: 15 fluid ounces (11 kcal)

➤ Low-fat milk: 3 fluid ounces (29 kcal)

➤ Diet drinks with no calories: 5 fluid ounces (1 kcal)

➤ Juices, sports drinks, whole milk, or alcohol: 15 fluid ounces (213 kcal)

➤ Regular soft drinks: 20 fluid ounces (211 kcal)

The above consumption values are averages from a population of people who filled out forms to record their daily beverage intake. Many people today consume many more kcal in non-water beverages and at much higher volumes than these numbers. The overconsumption of beverages that deliver calories but few nutrients has been cited as a possible contributing factor to today's obesity trends.

Dehydration

Thirst is a signal that your cells are becoming dehydrated. This problem is quickly rectified by drinking water or other beverages. If dehydration continues, the body falls into a serious health problem that may go from being reversible to irreversible. If you have lost at least 2 percent of your body weight due to dehydration, these symptoms will occur:

➤ 2 percent body weight loss: Strong thirst, loss of appetite, discomfort

➤ 4 percent loss: Reduced movement, flushed skin, weariness, sleepiness, nausea, and irritability

➤ 6 percent loss: Stumbling and dizziness, headache, tingling in extremities, increased body temperature and respiratory rate

➤ 8 percent loss: Labored breathing, blue skin due to oxygen deprivation, incoherent speech, and mental confusion

➤ 10 percent loss: Muscle cramps, incapacitation, loss of balance, swollen tongue, delirium

➤ Greater than 10 percent loss: Risk of death due to failing kidneys, decreased blood volume, and high salt concentration in blood

Serious cases of dehydration have occurred in endurance athletes, soldiers in training, and hikers and others who run out of water in the wilderness. People suffering from severe dehydration must see a medical provider immediately. Treatment includes intravenous fluid replacement, usually with a 5 percent glucose solution in water.

Nutrition Morsels

Most people know some of the health risks of dehydration but have no idea that too much water can be deadly too. Water intoxication results from consuming too much water so quickly that the kidneys cannot eliminate the excess. (Intoxication is the consumption of any substance at levels so high the substance becomes toxic or damaging to the body.) Consuming several quarts in a day or even within a shorter period causes sodium levels to fall too low. This affects various functions in the nervous system. Blurred vision is an early sign of water intoxication. Other symptoms are nausea, vomiting, confusion, disorientation, and possible seizures, coma, and/or death.

Water and Exercise

Thirst is your body's built-in safety mechanism for ensuring you never run dry. Intense physical exercise or labor raises your metabolic rate. To break down all those carbohydrates, fats, and perhaps proteins you need for energy, your cells need water molecules. Therefore, water intake should always be increased before and during strenuous activities or even moderately strenuous activities if done in hot weather.

Athletes (including dancers and physical laborers) need more water to keep cool and run their metabolism. Athletes should never allow their body to lose more than 2 percent of its weight in fluids excreted during exercise. For every 1 pound lost, a person should drink 2.5–3 cups of water during exercise or immediately afterward—the rule of thumb is 2 cups per pound.

To prevent dehydration during athletic activity, follow these guidelines:

➤ Drink as much water or diluted juice (diluted about 50:50 with water) as comfortable for the twenty-four-hour period before the activity.

➤ Drink 2 cups of water about 2 hours before the activity.

➤ For events lasting more than thirty minutes, drink about 1 cup every twenty minutes or every fifteen minutes in hot weather.

➤ Within four to six hours after exercise, drink 2.5–3 cups for every pound lost.

Most athletes know that if you feel thirsty, you are already dehydrated!

Nutrition Morsels

Drinking caffeine-containing beverages and beverages marketed as sports drinks has become increasingly popular for athletes and nonathletes who want an extra boost of energy when they hydrate. Each beverage has benefits and drawbacks.

Caffeine energy drinks (Monster, Red Bull, No Fear, Rockstar, and Full Throttle) contain about 100 milligrams of caffeine. Caffeine can increase alertness and provides a feeling of having extra energy, which may benefit an athlete during competition. But excessive caffeine consumption can lead to shakiness, anxiety, nausea, and insomnia in some people, and increases urination in everyone. Overall, the benefits of caffeine for athletic competition may be modest.

Sports drinks' claim to fame rests on the slug of sugars (usually several different forms) and electrolytes they give you. Sports drinks can contain up to 8 percent sugar. Since your body needs sugar and minerals for proper energy metabolism, sports drinks would seem to be beneficial additions to your water. For short bursts of energy, however, the body usually has plenty of sugars and other nutrients stored and ready for use.

Nutritionists seldom recommend sports drinks for hydration because the drinks add empty calories. But in intense physical activity lasting more than an hour, the body begins running out of electrolytes and sugars. In these situations, sports drinks are better than water for hydrating and replacing electrolytes such as sodium and potassium.

CHAPTER 21

Putting It All Together

In this chapter you will test your skills of seeing the big picture of nutrition. Learning about each nutrient group separately can be difficult because the nutrient classes weave together like tapestry to build your metabolism. You cannot study nitrogen without learning about amino acids, and you cannot understand amino acids without examining proteins. Likewise, protein metabolism interrelates with carbohydrate and fat metabolism. None of these processes can operate without vitamins and minerals.

In previous chapters, I broke down nutrition to its components. Now we will build them all back together to make the whole body's metabolism. Realize too that metabolism, the buildup and breakdown of nutrients for energy, is but a smaller piece of a puzzle called physiology.

Few people sit down to a meal and say, "I need more lysine today" or "I've been feeling a little low on biotin lately." Your enzymes, hormones, and certain organs keep track of the details of nutrient gains and losses. All you must do is construct a healthy diet with the correct balance of nutrients. Your digestive tract, enzymes, hormones, spleen, hypothalamus, brain, and other players in metabolism will sort it all out to keep your body running.

Let's build the big picture of nutrition by starting with your nutritional status. After understanding and assessing nutritional status, you get a clearer picture of what happens in metabolism. Then, this chapter will examine the current recommendations for how to select a diet to meet your metabolism's needs.

Knowing Your Nutritional Status

Nutritional status is also called your nutritional state. Your status is your health related to your level of nutrition. A nutritionist or a physician can determine your nutritional status by examining five factors:

1. Physical measurements, such as your height, weight, body fat, bone density, circumferences, and age

2. Biochemical measurements, such as the level of certain nutrients or their by-products in blood and urine

3. Physical examination, determining heart rate, blood pressure, respiratory rate, and any signs of illness

4. Dietary analysis to determine the amounts and proportions of nutrients and calories you consume

5. Economic evaluation to determine the probability of having a balanced diet or a diet that does not meet minimum nutrient requirements

Types of Nutritional Status

Three different types of nutritional status occur in all people: desirable nutrition, undernutrition, and overnutrition.

Desirable nutrition is your target. This occurs when your body tissues get enough of all nutrients to properly run metabolism and the body has some extra nutrients stored away in case of an increased need. Nutrients are typically stored in the liver, adipose tissue, bone, and muscle.

Undernutrition occurs when your nutrient intake cannot meet the body's nutrient needs. Everyone can skip an occasional meal or even fast for longer periods. Undernutrition starts when the body's nutrient stores can no longer make up the difference between intake and demand. As one or a few nutrients go missing, a person may show no outward signs of undernutrition. This is termed a subclinical nutrient deficiency. Prolonged nutrient deficiency will, however, begin to produce symptoms of a deficiency disease. This is known as a clinical nutrient deficiency.

Overnutrition is the prolonged consumption of more nutrients than the body needs. Short periods of overnutrition are common and should not be cause for concern. The period from Thanksgiving through Super Bowl Sunday has become a typical period of overnutrition in many households in this country. But a longer period of overconsumption of particular nutrients can lead to nutrient toxicity. Nutrient toxicities happen most commonly with vitamin A and from a variety of mineral supplements. The overwhelmingly most common overconsumption in the United States, however, is an excess intake of calories, which can lead to obesity.

Nutrition Vocabulary

Physiology is the science of all the systems of living organisms and how these systems work together to sustain life. Physiology includes all the body systems, such as the nervous system, musculature, and digestive system. It also encompasses all the chemical systems in your body. For instance, the acid-base balance of your blood, the action of antibodies to fight infection, and the secretion of hormones, enzymes, sweat, and gastric juices are all part of your unique physiology.

How Proteins, Fats, and Carbohydrates Work Together

The body uses carbohydrates first for energy, then turns to fats, and then resorts to proteins for energy only after the first two have been used up. But all living organisms try to run their metabolism in the most efficient way possible. Using carbohydrates, fats, and proteins in the exact sequence mentioned above is not as efficient as operating a continuous set of reactions in which glycogen is breaking down or building up, adipose tissue is releasing some fat and depositing others, and protein is either bulking up or slimming down.

For immediate energy, you take glucose from the liver's glycogen stores and burn it in glycolysis for energy. For sustained energy needs, your body supplements the glucose with fats from adipose tissue. After getting some energy from glycolysis, the glucose carbons are burned completely in the Krebs cycle and energy is generated from the electron transport chain of respiration. Fats are fed into the Krebs cycle too and generate energy the same way.

Burning extra energy often means your metabolic rate will increase. You might in turn need to build more muscle. Cells will need to replicate at a higher than normal rate. For this you need more DNA and the lipids, enzymes, other proteins, and carbohydrates that go into building new cells. You'll need nitrogen. Your diet should contribute plenty, but in a pinch some proteins can break down and liberate amino acids. The nitrogen from amino acids goes into new nucleic acids and new protein; the extra carbons from amino acids get fed into energy-generating routes such as the Krebs cycle.

Most amino acids can be converted chemically into a compound that is part of the Krebs cycle. Amino acids that cannot do this get converted into pyruvate. The carbons from pyruvate then go through a couple of easy steps before also entering the Krebs cycle.

During any lull in strenuous activity, the body replenishes cells and energy stores. The liver never wants to run completely out of glycogen; no matter how starved you are for glucose, some small bits of glycogen will remain in liver cells. The same is true for adipose tissue. The body prefers to retain a basal level of adipose for insulation, protection of internal organs, and perhaps to sequester toxic chemicals.

Your body is therefore seldom in a state of total breakdown or complete bulking up. Rather, you might be building up large storage molecules in one place while breaking down others in another part of the body.

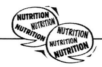

Nutrition Vocabulary

The terms *genesis* and *lysis* in nutrition tell you whether your body is building new cell materials or breaking them down. Gluconeogenesis is the production of new carbohydrate, specifically glucose. Lipogenesis is the building of new fats. Biochemists prefer the term *protein synthesis* to *proteogenesis*. When you break down these materials, your body operates glycolysis (glucose breakdown), lipolysis (fat breakdown), and proteolysis (protein breakdown). Therefore, genesis reactions are part of anabolism and lysis reactions are part of catabolism. They all work cooperatively to balance whole body metabolism.

Today's Nutrient Recommendations

The nutrient recommendations determined through research and published by the government are intended to keep an average, healthy person's metabolism in balance. That is, your anabolism and catabolism will work together to keep your cells healthy and energy stores stocked. At the same time, these processes will provide the energy you need to do normal daily activities. Of course, there is no such thing as an average person. Every individual has a specific lifestyle that may require tweaking the nutrient recommendations subscribed to by doctors and nutritionists.

Let's view the basic food groups that work best in supplying all the nutrients you need if you are an average person. In other words, these food groups in the right proportions add up to a balanced diet. For this discussion, an average person is an adult who is within the proper weight range for their height and age and has no chronic illnesses. At the end of this chapter I'll review the ways in which people often go off track in trying to assemble a balanced diet.

Nutrition Morsels

Obesity is a condition of having excess body fat. Obesity has been increasing in the United States since the 1960s. In 1962, 45 percent of adults between age twenty and seventy-five were overweight or obese. Today, about 65 percent of the population is overweight or obese.

Several factors contribute to today's obesity trend. The most likely factors are sedentary lifestyles, increases in total calorie intake, a shift in dietary norms to more energy-dense foods, and other behavioral factors.

Many nutrition resources offer height-weight charts that give you an idea if your weight is correct for your height or if you weigh too little or too much. Doctors and online resources can also calculate your body mass index (BMI), which is a measure of body fat based on height and weight. The BMI gives you an idea of whether your weight is appropriate for your height or outside the normal range. The BMI is discussed in more detail in the next chapter.

The Basic Food Groups

Does it seem like the basic food groups change every few years? Sometimes the government puts meat, dairy, vegetables, and carbohydrates into separate blocks in a diagram; sometimes nutritionists construct nutrients into an incomprehensible pyramid. Recently, the U.S. Department of Agriculture (USDA) introduced a new diagram for emphasizing the important food groups for balanced nutrition. It looks like a dinner plate with a portion each of protein foods, vegetables, grains, and fruits, with a cup of dairy on the side.

Will the USDA's MyPlate be the definitive guide on good nutrition into the distant future? Don't bet on it. Nutrition is a science; it changes as researchers gather new data, sift through facts and falsehoods, and confirm previous knowledge. Changes in nutrient recommendations do not mean that nutritionists don't know what they're doing. On the contrary, the changes indicate that nutrition experts are uncovering new information about how our body works and the roles played by nutrients in metabolism.

The Vegetable Group

In the USDA's dinner plate diagram, vegetables and grains each take up the largest portions. Together they provide complex carbohydrates, vitamins, and minerals with a minimum of fat, protein, and calories.

Vegetables should be varied by type and color to give you the best variety of the main nutrients supplied by each. In addition to being an excellent source of vitamins and minerals, vegetables increase your dietary fiber, which benefits you by controlling blood cholesterol and lowering the risk of heart disease, obesity, and type 2 diabetes. Vegetables are also high in water and low in calories.

Furthermore, you can meet your requirements for foods in the vegetable group by eating fresh, frozen, dried, cut, or pureed veggies.

The calories supplied by many vegetables are in the form of complex carbohydrates rather than sugars. Complex carbohydrates are digested more slowly and thus have a more moderate impact than sugars have on blood glucose levels following a meal. This helps keep your body in a steadier state of energy supply and demand than the sugar rush you might experience from other high-sugar foods.

The daily recommendations for vegetables are:

➤ Children up to eight years: 1–1.5 cups

➤ Boys and girls from nine to eighteen years: 2–3 cups

➤ Adults from nineteen to fifty years: 2.5–3 cups

➤ Adults over fifty years: 2–2.5 cups

In the above recommendations, boys and men usually require amounts at the higher end of the range, and older children require more than younger children in their age range. (See the USDA website for more details on all the food groups.)

The best vegetables for supplying a variety of vitamins and minerals with some fiber, complex carbohydrates, and water are:

➤ Dark green vegetables: Spinach, kale, broccoli, collard greens, turnip greens, watercress, bok choy, and dark leaf lettuce

➤ Red and orange vegetables: Carrots, acorn squash, butternut squash, sweet potatoes, tomatoes (usually categorized as a vegetable when cooking), red peppers, and tomato juice

➤ Starchy vegetables: Potatoes, corn, lima beans, and black-eyed peas

➤ Beans and peas: Beans (black, kidney, garbanzo, soy, pinto, white, and navy), lentils, and split peas

The Grains

Grains consist of two subgroups:

1. Whole grains: Made of the entire grain kernel (bran, germ, and endosperm) and include whole wheat flour, cracked wheat, oatmeal, rolled oats, whole cornmeal, quinoa, brown rice, wild rice, and popcorn (unbuttered)

2. Refined grains: Consist of only the kernel's endosperm and include white flour, white bread, tortillas (flour or corn), white rice, cornmeal, couscous, pasta, grits, and pretzels

Whole grains are good sources of fiber. Refined grains are poorer sources of fiber but because many have been fortified with vitamins and minerals, they are a good source of these nutrients.

Daily recommendations for grains are in ounce equivalents because grains come in a wide variety of shapes, sizes, and densities. To guide you, visualize one slice of bread or one half-cup of cooked rice or 1 cup of breakfast cereal (dry) as a single 1-ounce equivalent. With that picture imprinted on your mind, here are the daily recommendations for grains:

➤ Children up to eight years: 3–5-ounce equivalents

➤ Boys and girls from nine to eighteen years: 5–8-ounce equivalents

Nutrition Morsels

The ethanol in alcohol drinks yields about 7 kcal of energy per gram. Alcohol thus contributes to your overall energy balance but carries few other nutrients. For people with an alcohol abuse problem, consuming alcohol in place of nutrient-rich foods leads to numerous nutrient deficiencies.

Moderate consumption of alcohol by people of legal drinking age is not a health problem. Unfortunately, alcohol is often consumed at levels far higher than moderation. Although alcohol absorption by the body varies depending on gender, race, body size, and physical condition, and whether it is consumed with or without food, overconsumption leads to alcohol dependence, cirrhosis of the liver (loss of function of liver cells), coronary heart disease, disrupted sleep patterns, weakened immunity, and damage to nerves, bone, and muscles.

Most nutritionists define moderate alcohol use as about one drink per day for men and slightly less for women. The health risks described here begin to increase when consumption is more than about three drinks per day or binge drinking of more than four (women) or five (men) drinks in a short time period.

A standard drink is 12 ounces of beer, 5 ounces of wine, 3 ounces of a mixed drink (martini, whiskey sour, etc.), or 1.5 ounces of neat (straight) distilled liquors such as whiskey, brandy, cognac, rum, bourbon, gin, or vodka.

> ➤ Adults from nineteen to fifty years: 6–8-ounce equivalents

> ➤ Adults over fifty years: 5–6-ounce equivalents

The USDA also recommends that all people get a minimum level of grains each day. The minimum recommended amounts are about half of the daily recommendations shown above.

Nutrition Morsels

In the United States, the overall safety of our food supply is generally safe, meaning it contains few or no inorganic contaminants, such as toxic chemicals, or biological pests, such as microbes or insects. We owe this to rigorous food safety programs of the U.S. Department of Agriculture and the Food and Drug Administration. But even these large organizations cannot inspect every food item shipped from farms to table or imported from outside the U.S.

Some food ingredients are added intentionally to improve shelf-life, flavor, appearance, or other attributes that give food its attractiveness. Other things are in food unintentionally and may be a health hazard. Microbes and chemicals are the main contaminants of food. In some parts of the world, these contaminants spoil a limited food supply where people are already malnourished.

The main biological hazards in food are bacteria, molds, and insects. Foods can also contain viruses, protozoa, or toxins (poisons) made by some of these creatures. Many of the chemical contaminants in certain foods are environmental contaminants. This means the food is exposed to the chemicals during production and incorporates them into plant or animal tissue. When people eat these foods, they also ingest the environmental contaminants. Today's environmental food contaminants of the greatest concern are the metals cadmium, lead, and mercury, and the industrial chemicals dioxin, urethane, acrylamide, and polychlorinated biphenyls (PCBs).

The Proteins

The protein group used to be meat, eggs, and dairy products, with some beans to round out your amino acids supply. The revised recommendations now define the protein foods as meat, poultry, seafood, beans and peas, eggs, soy products, nuts, and seeds. It is important to eat a variety of these foods rather than focus on only one or two. Remember, every protein source has a limiting amino acid. To keep a steady and varied supply of amino acids coming into your cells' protein-building factories (called ribosomes), mix up your protein foods frequently. This food group is also an excellent source of B vitamins.

The daily recommendations for protein foods are:

> ➤ Children up to eight years: 2–4 ounces

> ➤ Boys and girls from nine to eighteen years: 5–6.5 ounces

> ➤ Adults from nineteen to fifty years: 5.5–6.5 ounces

> ➤ Adults over fifty years: 5–5.5 ounces

Read the package to get an idea of the size of an ounce of meat or poultry. For other foods, an ounce is about the size of one egg, 1 tablespoon of peanut butter, 0.25 cup cooked beans, or 0.5 cup of nuts or seeds.

Here are the foods that help you meet your protein requirements:

> ➤ Meat: Lean cuts of beef, veal, pork, ham, lamb, bison, venison, rabbit, calves' liver, and ground meats

> ➤ Poultry: Chicken, turkey, duck, goose, and ground poultry

> ➤ Seafood: Fish, shellfish, and canned fish

> ➤ Beans and peas: Beans (black, kidney, garbanzo, soy, pinto, white, and navy), lentils, and split peas

> ➤ Soy products: Tofu, soy veggie burgers, and tempeh

> ➤ Nuts: Almonds, cashews, peanuts, hazelnuts, walnuts, pecans, and pistachios

> ➤ Seeds: Pumpkin, sesame, and sunflower

When selecting from the seafood subgroup, try to focus on those that are good sources of omega-3 fatty acids. Examples are the fatty fishes such as salmon, trout, sardines, anchovies, herring, mackerel, and canned tuna.

The Fruit Group

As with vegetables, you can meet your requirements for foods in this group by eating fresh, frozen, dried, cut, or pureed varieties. Fruits are similar to vegetables as a good source of vitamins, minerals, complex carbohydrates, and water. Nutritionists recommend you eat a bit less fruits than vegetables because fruits tend to contain more sugar and less complex carbohydrates compared to vegetables.

Fruits are much better as snacks than candy, chips, cupcakes, or any other foods that we know as sweets. Fruits are also sweet, so they might satisfy your sweet tooth, but they provide a better variety of other nutrients than snack foods do.

The daily recommendations for fruits are:

> ➤ Children up to eight years: 1–1.5 cups

> ➤ Boys and girls nine to eighteen years: 1.5–2 cups

> ➤ Adults nineteen to fifty years: 1.5–2 cups

> ➤ Adults over fifty years: 1.5–2 cups

As a rule of thumb for putting together a balanced diet, try to get half your daily intake from the fruit and vegetable groups.

The best whole fruits for good nutrition are:

> ➤ Apples

> ➤ Pears

> ➤ Nectarines

> ➤ Citrus: Oranges, tangerines, lemons, limes, and grapefruit

> ➤ Berries: Strawberries, blueberries, raspberries, blackberries, loganberries, lingonberries, and olallieberries

> ➤ Bananas

> ➤ Plums

> ➤ Apricots

> ➤ Grapes

> ➤ Melons: Cantaloupes, honeydew melons, and watermelons

> ➤ Papayas

> ➤ Pineapples

> ➤ Mangoes

> ➤ Kiwifruit

Beware of fruits high in sugar and fairly low in complex carbohydrates (bananas, papayas, pineapples, mangoes, and kiwi fruit). Dried fruits such as prunes and raisins are good sources of fiber and berries supply antioxidants. Melons offer a great way to increase your water intake.

The Dairy Group

Foods from the dairy group supplement your protein intake and also supply good amounts of calcium, phosphorus, vitamin D, and riboflavin. Milk in whole, reduced fat (2 percent), low-fat (1 percent), or skim (fat-free) forms offers a wonderful way to hydrate while getting essential nutrients. Most brands of whole milk contain about 3.5 percent fat.

You should vary the foods you select from the dairy group as you vary those in all the other food groups. This helps you get the best blend of proteins, fats, and other essential nutrients.

People of all ages should try to limit their daily dairy food intake to not much more than 3 cups because some of these foods also contain a lot of fat. Look for low-fat or fat-free versions to help reduce fat intake.

To convert some of the dairy foods to a cup portion, use the following guidelines: 1 cup milk equals one slice of hard cheese (parmesan, mozzarella, or cheddar), one slice processed cheese (American), 2 cups of cottage cheese, or 1.5 cups of ice cream.

Foods that satisfy your dairy group requirements are:

➤ Milk: All fat-content varieties, flavored (chocolate or strawberry), and lactose-free or lactose-reduced

➤ Yogurt: All fat-content varieties

➤ Cheese: Hard, soft, and processed varieties

➤ Other dairy products: Ice cream, ice milk, frozen yogurt, and pudding made with milk

Oils

Oils are not a food group because they offer no nutrients except one, fat, which you can get from plenty of other foods. But nutritionists recommend you get some oils in your diet to supply the good fats that help control blood cholesterol.

Good oils are rich in poly- and monounsaturated fats. These fats contribute to a healthy spectrum of fats in your bloodstream and tissues.

Your normal intake of cooking oil plus nuts, fish, and salad dressings might give you enough good oils so that you need not supplement your diet with oil. To get the most out of oils, focus on the following foods:

➤ Oils, especially olive, canola, sunflower, safflower, corn, peanut, soybean, and cottonseed

➤ Nuts

➤ Olives

➤ Fish, especially the fatty fish in the protein foods group

➤ Avocados

Nutrition Morsels

We eat for energy, but for good nutrition we should make the best choices possible. The following four foods or nutrients are key for any energy-boosting diet:

1. Complex carbohydrates

2. Plant oils high in polyunsaturated fats

3. The recommended amounts of lean protein sources

4. Water

If you still need an energy boost from time to time, a cup of coffee is perfectly acceptable!

Avoid fats that are solid at room temperature (as opposed to liquid). Fats such as butter, lard, margarine, shortening, meat or poultry fats, and partially hydrogenated oils raise your bad lipoprotein levels in blood and lower the good lipoproteins. This is because they are high in saturated and trans fats.

In general, plant oils are better sources of fats than animal oils. But watch out for some exceptions. The plant oils from palm and coconut have high levels of saturated fats, so these two oils should be avoided too.

Where We Go Wrong

Balancing a diet isn't always easy if your lifestyle steers you to restaurants, fast-food joints, or the vending machine. Even people with the best intentions of choosing a healthy diet can be intimidated by the pressures of long workdays and short funds. Sometimes stopping at a fast-food restaurant is simply easier to face than stopping by the grocery and rattling pots and pans. These are the ways people make mistakes in their food choices:

➤ Too many calories for the level of physical activity

➤ Too many sugars and/or carbohydrates

➤ Too few foods supplying fiber and/or complex carbohydrates

➤ Too little water consumption

➤ Too much salt consumption

➤ Too many soft drinks and sweets instead of fruits and vegetables

➤ Too many refined grains instead of whole grains

➤ Too many processed foods in place of fresh vegetables and fruits

➤ Too many energy-dense foods (potato chips, cookies, mayonnaise, and butter) instead of nutrient-dense foods (lean meats, low-fat milk and yogurt, oranges, broccoli, and whole wheat breads and cereals)

Overhauling an entire diet may feel a bit like redoing your entire lifestyle. For the best success in developing a better balanced diet, tackle one food group at a time and make it part of your eating habits before focusing on the next goal.

CHAPTER 22

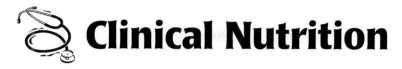 Clinical Nutrition

In this chapter you are introduced to the science of clinical nutrition and how it affects your dietary choices. This chapter focuses on the same topics that concern today's clinical nutritionists: the obesity problem and malnutrition. One of the true paradoxes of science lies in these two aspects of nutrition. While many people in the world are overweight and trending toward obesity, hunger is a constant torment to other populations. The majority of studies in clinical nutrition focus on these two disparate topics.

Who Are Clinical Nutritionists?

Clinical nutritionists study the science of how nutrients are digested, absorbed, transported, metabolized, stored, and eliminated, all in relation to maintaining good health.

Studies done by clinical nutritionists determine what nutrients we need, in what amounts, and the factors that might interfere with nutrient use. Clinical nutritionists also gather data on certain substances that may not be classified as nutrients, yet these substances contribute to improved health in specific ways. For example, clinical nutrition studies are underway in the following areas:

> ➤ Effects of eating fish during early pregnancy to protect against early delivery and underweight babies

> ➤ The role of vitamin E in specific heart ailments

> ➤ Folate's role in potentially lowering the risk of stroke or heart disease

> ➤ Carotenoids for reducing the risk of cataracts

> ➤ Carotenoids and flavonoids for protecting against cancers

Studies on many additional topics are also taking place in clinical nutrition departments at universities. In addition to adding to our total knowledge of nutrients and nutrition, clinical nutritionists are always working to uncover changing trends in nutrition. This includes the promising trends, such as the increased understanding that the North American diet has long needed more fiber in it. Of more immediate concern are trends indicating that people are in nutritional trouble, which could soon threaten their health.

Weight and Obesity

Nutritionists have devised a calculation for determining if a person is at their ideal weight with an appropriate amount of body fat, or if they are outside their ideal range. Called the body mass index (BMI), this measurement tells you if you are dangerously low in body stores of fat and other nutrients or dangerously overstocked. The BMI is available in printed charts or online calculators. All you need to know is your height and weight.

The BMI calculation is simply body weight divided by height, with a conversion factor thrown in to adjust to metric values. For example, a person weighing 150 pounds and standing 5 feet 8 inches tall would have a BMI value of 23. The chart or calculator then tells you what your value means according to these guidelines:

> ➤ Underweight: Less than 18.5

> ➤ Normal weight: 18.5–24.9

> ➤ Overweight: 25.0–29.9

> ➤ Obese: 30 or greater

People with a BMI of 40 or greater are greatly risking their health. The condition is called severe obesity or morbid obesity. While being severely obese was once a rarity associated mainly with physiological disorders, an alarming number of Americans enter this category every year because they take in many more calories than they burn with physical activity. The trend does not show any signs of slowing.

The BMI is a guideline only. It does not take into account a person's gender or age and does not account for any underlying illness.

Anyone who is overweight to obese has a higher risk of health problems:

> ➤ Type 2 diabetes: Enlarged adipose cells stuffed with fat do not respond well to insulin for controlling blood glucose.

> ➤ Cardiovascular disease: Increased blood levels of LDL and fats (triglycerides) occlude blood vessels. Other factors, such as an increase in blood clotting mechanisms and release of inflammatory factors in the blood put added stress on the heart.

> ➤ Hypertension: The dramatic increase in the number of blood vessels that serve the enlarged adipose tissue makes normal blood pressure impossible.

> ➤ Hormonal imbalance: Estrogen produced by adipose cells increases the risk of cancers and makes pregnancy and delivery difficult.

> ➤ Liver damage: Excess fat accumulation in the liver interferes with normal function.

> ➤ Erectile dysfunction: Excess fat lining the blood vessels decreases the male's sexual performance.

> ➤ Pulmonary disease: Excess weight on the lungs and pharynx reduce breathing efficiency.

> ➤ Impaired vision: Obesity increases the incidence of cataracts and other eye disorders

In addition to the above risks, overweight people are more difficult to do surgery on because of adjustments to anesthesia, extra adipose surrounding internal organs, and a greater risk of wound infections.

Nutrition Morsels

The best way to lose weight is to decrease calorie intake while increasing calorie output through physical activity. You will not gain weight if you use up in activity about the same amount of calories you consume, whether the intake is 1,500 kcal, 2,500 kcal, or 4,000 kcal. If you only eat 1,500 kcal a day but sit at your computer all day burning off about 1,000 kcal, you'll gain weight. Similarly, you can eat as much as 4,000 kcal a day and still lose weight if you're also burning up 5,000 kcal in exercise. No magic formula exists for losing weight, and there never will be a magic formula. To lose weight, eat less and exercise more!

Weight and Malnutrition

In destitute areas of the United States and many other parts of the world, undernutrition is a far greater problem than overnutrition. About 2 billion people in the world experience some sort of food shortage every day. This number is probably an underestimate of the crisis. Indigenous people on the outskirts of society, the homeless, and those displaced by natural disasters and war tend not to be counted by even the most intrepid researchers.

The two main types of undernutrition are hunger and malnutrition. Hunger is the strong sensation of needing something to eat. Malnutrition is any impairment to normal metabolism because of a deficiency (or excess) of one or more nutrient. Malnutrition caused by deficiencies can become severe enough to turn into hunger. If hunger persists, starvation follows.

The leading chronic problem in many societies is protein-calorie malnutrition (PCM). In PCM, a person does not get their required daily amount of calories or protein. Some malnutrition diseases—kwashiorkor and marasmus discussed in Chapter 27—arise from PCM.

Nutritionists have identified several nutrients that are deficient in many places worldwide, even in wealthy nations. These nutrients are:

➤ Iron

➤ Zinc

➤ Vitamin A

➤ Iodide

➤ Various B vitamins, especially B12, thiamin, and niacin

Why don't we solve such easily identifiable nutrition problems? Part of the reason is political. Organizations have trouble crossing international boundaries to rescue people who are starving, hungry, or malnourished. Nutrition is often connected to politics, even in the United States as you will see later in this chapter.

Nutrition Morsels

Part of a clinical nutritionist's job is to figure out the variety and amounts of nutrients to keep a body in a state called homeostasis. Homeostasis is a condition in which a body maintains its internal equilibrium by constantly adjusting to the external environment. All body systems take part in homeostasis, but it is led mainly by your sensory, nervous, and circulatory systems, and by hormones from the endocrine system.

Clinical Trials in Human Nutrition

A clinical trial is a carefully designed study of the effects of a substance on a large number of human volunteers. In nutrition, clinical trials on a particular disease might include one hundred or more people.

In nutrition, clinical trials often test the effects of a nutrient in correcting the symptoms of a disease. These clinical trials must use volunteers who already have a certain identified disease. The clinical researchers then collect data from the volunteers over a long time period to determine if the nutrient is correcting the disease symptoms and if there are other signs related to nutritional status.

Researchers also conduct similar studies called field trials. These studies are conducted on much larger groups of volunteers, from several hundred to thousands. Field trials study the effects of a dietary substance on healthy volunteers.

Animal Studies in Human Nutrition

Animals have been used in studies on human nutrition when the study design is too difficult or too dangerous to be conducted on people. Rats, mice, and rabbits have been used for evaluating lipoprotein effects on tissue, the physiology of severe obesity, and gene therapy related to nutrient use.

Most feeding experiments using animals are known to be of limited value for making conclusions about human nutrition. They, nevertheless, are useful in determining whether a nutrient is needed for a living organism.

Getting to a Recommended Daily Allowance

The recommended dietary allowance (RDA) is also called a dietary reference standard. By either name, it equals the nutrient intake in an amount sufficient to meet the needs of about 98 percent of people in a certain age range.

The RDAs for all the essential nutrients we now recognize have been determined through of combination of methods:

➤ Deprivation studies: Removing the nutrient from the diet of an animal and observing any deficiency symptoms

➤ Balance studies: Comparison of the intake and excretion of a nutrient to determine if the body is accumulating it or eliminating an excess

➤ Radioactive tracer studies: Putting a radioactively labeled nutrient in the food and analyzing its movement into tissue and excretion

> ➤ Biological tissue studies: Measuring the amount of nutrient needed to maintain a certain level in blood or tissue

> ➤ Biological markers: Measuring the activity of a certain tissue or organ known to be dependent on a given nutrient

> ➤ Biochemical markers: Measuring secretions from a certain tissue or organ known to be dependent on a given nutrient

Fighting Disease with Clinical Nutrition

Proper nutrition can fight certain diseases as long as the disease is caused by a nutrient imbalance and not infection or genetics. Clinical nutritionists know that certain non-nutrition-related health conditions can influence nutrient use.

The following conditions cannot be cured with proper nutrition alone, but a balanced diet is key for successful treatment:

> ➤ Biological conditions: Tobacco addiction, alcohol addiction, hypertension, and obesity

> ➤ Noncommunicable diseases: Cardiovascular diseases (atherosclerosis, stroke, vascular disease, heart attack, lung disease, diabetes, osteoporosis, cirrhosis, diet-induced cancers, and dental caries

> ➤ Behavioral conditions: Smoking, alcohol abuse, sedentary lifestyle, and any dietary imbalance

The World Health Organization's RDAs

The WHO has compiled the results from thousands of studies using the methods listed above. It has published goals for adults for preventing death or disability from nutrient-related diseases. These RDAs for nutrients or foods are:

> ➤ Protein: 10–15 percent of total energy intake

> ➤ Total carbohydrate: 55–75 percent of total energy

> ➤ Sugars: Not more than 10 percent of total energy

> ➤ Total fat: 15–30 percent of total energy

> ➤ Saturated fatty acids: Not more than 10 percent of total energy

> ➤ Polyunsaturated fatty acids: 6–10 percent of total energy

> ➤ Omega-6 polyunsaturated fatty acids: 5–8 percent of total energy

➤ Omega-3 polyunsaturated fatty acids: 1–2 percent of total energy

➤ Cholesterol: Not more than 300 milligrams per day

➤ Sodium chloride: Not more than 5 grams per day

➤ Non-starch polysaccharides: More than 20 grams per day

➤ Total fiber: More than 25 grams per day

➤ Fruits and vegetables: At least 400 grams per day

Why Nutrition Information Keeps Changing

RDAs change over time when new data on nutrient requirements replace obsolete data. But not all nutrition recommendations are based solely on scientific data; the human food supply is regulated by government. Government can be influenced by special interest groups. When U.S. political action committees (PACs) and industry organizations represent food producers, the RDAs for the American public might be influenced.

The list below shows some of today's food industry organizations that have a vested interest in the amount of protein, eggs, dairy, and other foods the USDA recommends for good health. Many of these groups are nonprofit associations that represent their industry's interests in Washington, DC, when new legislation is proposed for crop prices, trucking regulations, pollution, and nutritional recommendations for humans. Some focus less on legislation and more on science-based recommendations for human nutrition. All have information on the particular food groups they represent.

➤ American Meat Producers Association

➤ American Sheep Industry Association

➤ International Dairy Foods Association

➤ National Broiler Council

➤ National Cattlemen's Beef Association

➤ National Dairy Council

➤ National Fisheries Institute

➤ National Pork Producers Council

➤ National Turkey Federation

➤ United Fresh Produce Association

➤ U.S. Poultry and Egg Association

Many additional national and state organizations can be found that represent regional food producers, such as the Idaho Potato Commission. In addition, you can find specialty groups that concentrate on a particular food, such as the National Peach Council, the American Dairy Goat Association, or the National Yogurt Association. If there is a food you're interested in learning more about, there is probably an organization representing it and offering good information on its nutrition.

The U.S. Department of Agriculture acts as this country's national organization for all agricultural products made in the United States as well as imported products.

Despite the uneasy mixing of politics and nutrition, almost everyone's goal inside and outside of government is the correct nutrient recommendations for a healthy population. Although it seems as if politics and money sometimes lead us astray, over time our nutritional recommendations always return to science-based facts from clinical nutrition studies.

PART SIX

Nutrition Choices and Health

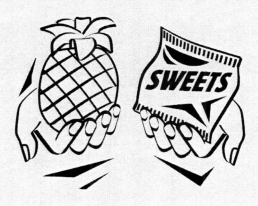

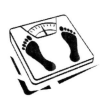

CHAPTER 23

Losing or Gaining Weight: How to Fix Energy Imbalance

In This Chapter

➤ Safe methods for gaining or losing weight

➤ Energy outputs of various physical activities

➤ Strategies and tips for weight control programs

In this chapter you learn the safest and most nutritionally sound ways to lose weight or gain weight. Perhaps no other aspect of nutrition is as fraught with error as the do-it-yourself weight loss or weight gain plan. This chapter shows you how to reach your weight loss or weight gain goals by following the same principles of good nutrition described elsewhere in this book.

This chapter presents no magic formulas or nutrition secrets! In fact, if you ever hear the words *foolproof*, *fantastic*, or *fast* to describe a weight loss or weight gain program, run the other way! Even the word *fun* to describe weight programs makes me nervous—if it was fun, wouldn't we all be the perfect weight?

The recommendations in this chapter are for those seeking to lose or gain from 7 to 35 pounds. Many people's weight fluctuates in a range of 5 to 7 pounds over several months, so we won't worry about fine-tuning body weight within that range. For people who need to lose or gain more than 35 pounds, I advise you first check with your family physician. In fact, any weight program should be discussed with your doctor, a trained nutritionist, or a registered dietician before you begin. Your physician will be aware of any underlying health conditions that might affect nutrient and energy balance as well as interactions of nutrients with any medications you take. The severely undernourished or the obese require special medical attention for tackling a weight adjustment program in the safest possible way.

Balancing Energy Intake and Output

As mentioned in the previous chapter, weight fluctuations can be distilled to a simple equation. Mind your energy inputs and outputs, and you will be able to control your weight; increase it, decrease it, or stay the same. These are the energy balance equations:

> ➤ Weight gain: Kcal in are greater than kcal out
> ➤ Weight loss: Kcal in are less than kcal out

Energy (kcal) intake comes from the diet. You can count up the amount of calories on this half of the equation by reading the label on the food's packaging or looking up a food, such as an apple, in a nutrition book or online.

Energy output equals the amount of kcal your body uses up in metabolism. Energy output is harder to put a number on. Some energy is spent in digesting, absorbing, and transporting foods and nutrients in the body. Normal resting metabolism also burns some kcal. These are relatively small energy outputs compared with the energy burned in physical activity. So while resting metabolism helps burn away some calories, to really move fat off your body you will need to increase your physical activity. For those of you trying to gain weight, increasing the body's bulk in the form of muscle and bone mass also relates to a regimen of physical exercise.

Few things in biology work as well together as good nutrition and a sound physical exercise program.

Energy Output

Increasing physical activity means turning off the TV and getting on a bicycle, stepping away from the keyboard and taking a walk, or turning over the garden instead of leafing through cheesecake recipes. If your BMI is 25 or higher, you need to increase your energy output to be higher than energy intake.

For the first phase of your weight loss/gain program, you may want to keep track of kcal in and kcal out to get an idea of your personal energy balance equation. Once you have a feel for your average input and output, you may not need to calculate the totals every day. Examples of energy output activities for a 150-pound person are:

➤ Running about 9 minutes/mile: 250 kcal/20 minutes; 750 kcal/1 hour

➤ Bicycling about 15 mph: 227 kcal/20 minutes; 682 kcal/1 hour

➤ Aerobics, 6–8-inch step: 193 kcal/20 minutes; 580 kcal/1 hour

➤ Basketball game, playing: 182 kcal/20 minutes; 545 kcal/1 hour

➤ Elliptical trainer: 164 kcal/20 minutes; 491 kcal/1 hour

➤ Sweeping the garage: 91 kcal/20 minutes; 273 kcal/1 hour

➤ Vacuuming: 80 kcal/20 minutes; 239 kcal/1 hour

➤ Walking about 17 minutes/mile: 75 kcal/20 minutes; 259 kcal/1 hour

➤ Bowling: 68 kcal/20 minutes; 204 kcal/1 hour

➤ Watching bowling on TV: 23 kcal/20 minutes; 68 kcal/1 hour

The energy output values listed above account for basal metabolism plus the amount of energy needed to do the activity. Several online programs offer diet analysis calculators that help you keep track of all your inputs and outputs. The USDA website offers a free kcal tracker based on your weight for various physical activities.

Energy Output Efficiency

Few things feel as unbearable as when a person first begins an exercise program, and because of this the program often begins and ends on Day 1. But if you can stick with an exercise program that is reasonable for your age, weight, and health—check with your physician first!—the program becomes increasingly easier to maintain. This is because exercise improves the efficiency of body metabolism in various ways:

➤ Strengthens the heart so that oxygen and nutrients are pumped to the tissues more efficiently

➤ Increases blood vessel development in muscle and organs, further helping oxygen and nutrient delivery and waste removal

Nutrition Vocabulary

Resting metabolism is the amount of calories an awake body uses when a person has not eaten for about four hours. During this resting period, the body's organs burn some energy just to keep running. For example, the liver burns 380 kcal/day. Other resting organs or tissues burn the following amount of energy:

➤ Brain: 265 kcal/day

➤ Skeletal muscle: 250 kcal/day

➤ Kidneys: 140 kcal/day

➤ Heart: 100 kcal/day

➤ Various other tissues: 265 kcal/day

➤ Builds muscle, which aids blood circulation, especially the return of venous blood to the heart

➤ Strengthens bone, which enhances the calcium-phosphorus exchange with tissues

➤ Enhances enzyme systems involved in energy metabolism

➤ Enhances hormone secretion involved in mood and energy

➤ Reduces stress, thereby reducing hypertension and many inefficiencies of nutrient use

Nutrition Morsels

A registered dietician (RD) is a person who has met specific academic and professional requirements to advise the public on nutrition. A person must pass an exam administered by the American Dietetic Association to be called an RD. An RD is a nutritionist, that is, a person trained in human nutrition. Many people with academic training and a degree in nutrition are nutritionists, but only those nutritionists who have passed the required exam and met other professional requirements have earned the title of RD.

Weight Loss Strategies

The safest approach to a successful weight loss program is to go slowly and steadily with the understanding that an occasional mistake does not undermine all your previous progress. Here are useful guidelines for planning a weight loss program:

➤ Set your goals with the help of a physician or trained nutritionist.

➤ Plan a program that depends on both reduced calorie intake and increased physical activity.

➤ Target achievable increments of reduced calorie intake, for example, decreasing intake by 100 kcal every one to three days.

➤ Do the same slow, steady increase in physical activity by increasing daily energy output by about 100 kcal every one to three days.

➤ Control total calorie intake rather than eliminate any of the five recommended food groups. Make sure you meet your minimum nutrient requirements for everything except energy.

➤ Build in a reward or a free day. Within reason (one scoop of ice cream instead of three), give yourself a treat once week.

➤ Eliminate the energy-dense foods that you didn't like much anyway. If you don't like mayonnaise, an easy way to rid your diet of its calories is to stop eating it. You won't miss it anyway.

Although physical activity is important in any weight loss program, your attention should always go first to calorie intake. Snacking on even healthy foods adds to total daily intake, and many people snack for reasons that have nothing to do with appetite:

➤ Boredom

➤ Anxiety

➤ Depression

➤ Social pressures

➤ "Because it's there"

Tips to Keeping a Weight Loss Program on Track

Eating and behavior are tied together in western society. We eat to be social, polite, and to keep our hands (and mouth) busy in uncomfortable situations. Nutritionists have devised several tactics that help control an overweight person's behavior related to food. The National Weight Control Registry has a more extensive list of tips. Here are some of the tips I find most useful:

➤ Eat breakfast: Breakfast takes care of mid-morning snack cravings and provides the energy needed to last until lunch.

➤ Try to exercise about one hour per day: If you have a time crunch in your schedule, you can add exercise to whatever total you achieve by taking stairs instead of the elevator, walking your dog (or your neighbor's!), parking as far from the mall entrance as possible, and jogging, rather than walking, at home to complete simple tasks.

➤ Do grocery shopping after eating: Shop from a list and emphasize fresh foods, avoiding ready-to-eat packaged foods.

➤ Keep snack foods out of sight or lock them up: Eat meals and snacks only in designated places, such as the kitchen or work cafeteria.

➤ Use smaller dishes and always try to leave some food (calories) on the plate: Put the fork down between mouthfuls and pause for a moment in the middle of each meal.

➤ Pack a healthy lunch for work: Try to limit restaurant meals (including fast food) to not more than twice a week.

➤ At fast food restaurants, order the kid's meal.

➤ Eat smart at fast-food restaurants: Many fast food restaurants charge more money for ordering à la carte. To save money while sparing calories, order the meal, then fill your soda cup with water instead of a soft drink, and throw away half the fries or substitute salad for fries. (When you get good at this you may decide to discard all the fries!)

➤ Get doggie bags at restaurants: In restaurants that serve large portions—many restaurant meals exceed entire daily calorie allotments—eat until you're no longer hungry and bring the leftovers home for the next day. You can even ask your server to put half your entrée into a container before bringing the meal to your table.

➤ Watch the size of portions: Order a cup of soup instead of a bowl. You can also substitute appetizers or small plates (tapas) for a full entrée. Never supersize anything!

➤ Stick to the rules of a balanced diet with adequate fiber and limited fat even when eating meals away from home.

Weight Gain Strategies

If your BMI is less than 18.5 and you have no chronic or acute disease, cancer, or digestive system disorders, you probably need to gain weight. Being too underweight is a health risk associated with the following:

➤ Bone loss

➤ Slow recovery from illness

➤ Difficulty in pregnancy or delivery

➤ Abnormal menstrual cycles

➤ Poor storage of fat-soluble nutrients

➤ Disrupted hormone function

➤ Poor thermoregulation (regulation of body temperature)

➤ Inadequate energy for normal activities

The underweight condition has not been studied in North America as much as factors related to being overweight or obese. Obesity appears to be a greater concern and a faster emerging trend. Also, being underweight is often socially acceptable as evidenced by emaciated-looking fashion models and celebrities.

In growing children with very high levels of physical activity and play, being underweight is a common occurrence. Growth spurts in adolescents also contribute to being underweight.

The most successful weight gain strategies incorporate some or all of the following:

➤ Adhere to a regular meal and snack schedule.

➤ Make meals a priority in your schedule.

➤ Eat at least the minimum daily recommendations for fat and carbohydrates.

➤ Use a physical exercise program that builds muscle mass and strengthens bones, such as weight lifting. In general, replace endurance sports (distance running, long-distance cycling, triathlons) with strength sports (power lifting, gymnastics, hiking, water polo, rowing and kayaking, slow dancing, yoga).

➤ If you are excessively active, reduce physical activity by skipping the gym, workouts, or other training once or twice a week.

➤ Target an extra 500 kcal per day relative to energy output by either eating more or exercising less.

Set Point

Does the body have a set point, that is a body weight or fat content it is genetically predetermined to reach? Nutritionists have long debated the role of the set point in weight control or even if set point truly exists.

Set point remains a theory. Nutrition researchers know the body has mechanisms for maintaining homeostasis. Hunger and satiety are obvious aspects of weight control. To conserve energy, certain glands and hormones activate when energy (calorie) intake decreases and metabolism slows. Adipose tissue is furthermore programmed to protect the body against weight loss more than weight gain. Thus, it is easier to gain weight than to lose it.

Despite knowing the body has mechanisms to help regulate weight, a set point for the body, for adipose tissue, or for the number of fat cells you have in your body has never been proven.

Tips for a Successful Weight Program

The types and amounts of food we eat have long ago been disconnected from the need to simply fuel metabolism. If you are embarking on a plan to adjust your weight, you'll need to overcome certain obstacles that society and your own behavioral tendencies throw in your way. Keep these things in mind if you are seeking to lose weight, gain weight, or even stay right where you are:

➤ Never be ashamed of your weight: It's not against the law to be under- or overweight. Your weight adjustment plan should be for you, your health, and no one else.

➤ Start mid-month rather than on January 1st: A first-of-the-year start date puts a spotlight on how far you've come and how far you still have to go on a diet program. Take the pressure off yourself by picking another date in a different month.

➤ Tell your friends or tell no one: Some people enjoy the support and encouragement of friends on a shared quest to get to the perfect weight. To others, all that encouragement can feel more like nagging. Pick the approach that is right for you. There are no wrong ways to do it.

➤ Relapse happens: A nutritionist will give you tips on how to avoid going astray during your control program. But occasional lapses occur and they do not mean you have failed. Don't overreact to mistakes. Figure out a way to avoid or minimize future lapses and take credit for acknowledging it and planning to do better in the future.

➤ Keep a journal, or not: Some people have more success if they record their daily intake. Others find this task annoying and enough to make them drop their program altogether. Personality is a big part of your relationship with food, so do what you know works best for you.

➤ Any exercise is better than no exercise: Don't be hard on yourself if you stayed late at work all week and could not squeeze in a daily hour at the gym. Did you manage to squeeze in twenty minutes on Monday? Did you substitute a workout with a brisk walk around the block? Good. Keep going. Tomorrow always brings another chance to get it right.

➤ It's not a race: Avoid comparing yourself to others on similar weight programs. Your physiology is unique to you. Rid yourself of statements like, "I'll never look as good as she does," "Compared to him, I look fine," or "I can cheat a little and still weigh less than her."

➤ Pay attention to how you feel during a meal: Stop eating when you no longer feel hungry. Period.

Nutrition Morsels

Why does the United States have an obesity problem and why is it spreading to other parts of the world? Obesity can come either from genetic or environmental causes. The amount of fat stored in a person's body and the main places in the body where it gets stored are inherited. Basal metabolism rate is also inherited. If you have inherited a slightly slower than normal metabolic rate, you might have a tendency to gain weight. If you have a slightly faster basal metabolic rate, you might have a hard time keeping weight on your body. Our genes may contribute up to 70 percent of the weight differences between people.

Many environmental causes have exaggerated the genetic predisposition to be overweight. These environmental reasons for weight gain have led to an increasingly overweight population and have also increased the percentage of people defined as obese. Some of the main environmental factors believed to contribute to our overweight problem are:

➤ Jobs that demand less physical exertion and more sedentary activity

➤ Increased reliance on energy dense (high-fat, high-calorie) diets

➤ Size acceptance

CHAPTER 24

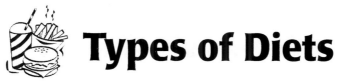

Types of Diets

> ## In This Chapter
>
> ➤ Hallmarks of all healthy diets
> ➤ Types of vegetarian diets
> ➤ Special diets for pregnancy, training, and aging
> ➤ How to spot fad diets

In this chapter you will become acquainted with the different types of diets most common in our society. Any of these diets can provide good nutrition, but some have pitfalls. This chapter examines the advantages and disadvantages of each. If you want to change your diet, after reading this chapter you'll know the reasons why certain diets work for particular nutrition circumstances.

Considering that hundreds of different diets are touted in cookbooks, on TV, and on websites, it seems impossible to separate the wheat from the chaff, or the safe and healthy from the unsafe. This chapter cannot cover all the diets now being tried or emerging almost weekly, but it will help you focus on the hallmarks of all safe and healthy diets.

The Hallmarks of All Healthy Diets

All healthy diets have the following characteristics:

> ➤ A balance of nutrients and the recommended food groups that supply them
> ➤ At least two daily servings of fruit and three daily servings of vegetables, with at least one-third being dark green or deep yellow vegetables

➤ At least six daily servings of grain products, with at least three servings being whole grains

➤ Less than 5 grams of salt

➤ Foods that minimize the intake of cholesterol, saturated fats, and trans fats

➤ Alcohol consumption no greater than recommended limits

➤ A minimum intake of energy-dense foods and an emphasis on nutrient-dense foods

How to Spot Unhealthy Fad Diets

A fad diet (also called a novelty diet) is any diet currently popular with the public without the universal backing of physicians and nutritionists. Some of these diets develop into acceptable programs for meeting certain nutritional goals, but many lead to more health problems the longer a person sticks with the diet. In other words, some diet fads are worse than others.

Make sure any diet you consider meets all of the criteria listed above. Seek advice about the diet from a physician or trained nutritionists before beginning on it. Read about the diet also on your own. A fad diet will have at least one of the following features:

➤ Emphasizes one food group or one nutrient more than others or to the exclusion of all other nutrients. Examples are low-carbohydrate (low-carb), low-fat, high-protein, or high-fiber diets. These diets can be beneficial for weight control and some chronic diseases if you follow them under a doctor's or nutritionist's care. Trouble usually occurs when a diet calls for severe restrictions that cause nutrient imbalance. The Atkin's Diet, Zone Diet, and South Beach Diet belong in this category, although none of these examples are restrictive to the point of being unhealthy. Other less desirable examples are the cabbage soup diet and the grapefruit diet.

➤ Focuses on restrictions, usually for losing weight. Most weight loss diets unsurprisingly target fat intake. Reducing dietary fat too much can decrease the absorption of fat-soluble nutrients. Severe restrictions are also difficult to maintain and increase your chances of failing to meet your nutritional goals. Examples of restrictive diets are the Pritikin Diet, the McDougall Program, the Rice Diet, and the Okinawa Program. The prominent weight loss programs (Weight Watchers and Jenny Craig) control total calorie intake while developing a balanced diet for their customers, which are safe and effective approaches to weight loss.

➤ Uses meal replacements. These diets depend on replacing one or more daily meals with a beverage, prepared entrée (frozen or self-stable), or a snack or energy bar. Slim-Fast is an example of this type of diet.

➤ Makes unrealistic claims. These diets may be easiest to spot by their names. They claim improbable results in time periods that seem illogical. Examples are the 3-Hour Diet, the Fat Smash Diet, and the Fit for Life Diet. Others in this group imply they are successful based on their geographical use: the Beverly Hills Diet or the New Hilton Head Metabolism Diet. With respects to the Garden State, these diets sound a bit more appealing than the New Jersey Swamplands Diet, don't they?

The best way to ensure safety and success is to understand the disadvantages of fad diets and avoid them altogether or modify them to maintain good nutrition. For example, the following modifications should be considered for each group of fad diet described above:

➤ Diets that emphasize one food group or nutrient: Maintain a balanced diet even while emphasizing one food or nutrient. Make sure to meet all nutrient RDAs and not exceed any upper limits known for some vitamins and minerals. Pay attention to any symptoms of nutrient imbalance: headaches, muscle cramps, constipation, and halitosis (bad breath).

➤ Restrictive diets: Follow only under the supervision of a physician who may prescribe appropriate vitamin and mineral supplements.

➤ Meal replacement diets: Follow only under the supervision of a physician who may prescribe appropriate vitamin and mineral supplements and will monitor vegetable, fruit, and fiber intake.

➤ Diets making outlandish claims: Avoid. These diets lead to malnutrition faster than the others and their consequences can be damaging to the body.

Nutrition Morsels

Why do fad diets succeed, at least in the short-term? Many people are desperate to lose weight and have not had success with the slow, steady approach to weight control. Fad diets sometimes offer astounding results in a short amount of time with little to no exercise required! For people wanting to make a quick buck off the frustration of others, rolling out a new diet with little scientific credence is tempting.

Testimonials from people who have succeeded on the diet often make matters worse. By luck or good timing, these people have had success on a fad diet and recommend it to their friends. The friends then give it a try rather than checking in with their doctor or doing the appropriate amount of research on the diet's claims.

The best sources for doing due diligence on a diet that interests you are scientific journals and universities with a human nutrition department. Stick to journals that publish only peer-reviewed articles: the *Journal of the American Medical Association*, *The New England Journal of Medicine*, the *Journal of the American Dietetic Association*, and the *Journal of Nutrition*.

Watch out for any new diet that promotes quick weight loss, claims to cure certain diseases, severely limits food selections, demands that one food (for example, grapefruit or cabbage soup) substitute for a meal, requires expensive supplements, or gives no guidance on overall nutrition or eating habits.

For example, a diet asking you to eat nothing but saltine crackers for a month will undoubtedly allow some weight loss. But what happens after the month is up? Does the diet give you further advice on weight maintenance or tell you that you may now return to your normal eating habits?

The two biggest warning signs of a fad diet are:

1. Testimonials from movie stars

2. Claims that you do not need to exercise on this diet to lose weight

Vegetarian Nutrition

Vegetarian diets have been chosen by people for centuries for philosophical, religious, ethical, economic, and health reasons. For these same reasons, vegetarian diets have evolved into a variety of subgroups. Thus, merely describing yourself as vegetarian, a person who doesn't eat meat, no longer tells the whole story. The following list provides a glimpse of the many types of vegetarianism practiced today throughout the world:

➤ Vegetarian: A person who abstains from all animal foods, including meat, poultry, seafood, game, and animal by-products such as gelatin.

➤ Vegan: A person who abstains from all animal foods, all animal by-products, and all foods of animal origin, such as milk, eggs, and honey. That is, a person who eats only plant foods.

➤ Lactovegetarian: A person who consumes only plant foods and dairy products.

➤ Ovo-lactovegetarian (or lacto-ovo-vegetarian): A person who consumes only plant foods, dairy products, and eggs.

➤ Fruitarian: A person who eats mainly fruits, nuts, seeds, honey, and vegetable oils.

Advantages of Vegetarian and Vegan Diets

Vegetarian and vegan diets are heart-healthy diets. These diets lower blood cholesterol because they lack cholesterol, which comes only in animal foods. They are low in saturated and trans fat and, in fact, are usually low in total fats. Vegetarian and vegan diets also supply good amounts of fiber.

Vegetarian and vegan diets contain substances called phytochemicals, which have been associated with preventing certain types of cancers. Some doctors therefore promote these diets for patients with a history of breast, prostate, and colon cancer.

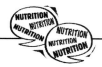

Nutrition Vocabulary

Phytochemicals are chemicals found in plants—the term *phyto* means "plant." Some phytochemicals have been suspected of reducing the risk of certain cancers in people who consume them regularly. A vast array of phytochemicals occur in your diet. These are:

➤ Carotenoids

➤ Sulfur-containing thiocyanates

➤ The fruit hormones daidzein, genistein, and isoflavones

➤ The seed hormone group coumestans

➤ Various plant antioxidants

Although phytochemicals have been increasingly credited with preventing cancers and reducing the number of cancer cells in people already diagnosed with cancer, we should remember that these chemicals are found throughout many diets. Many people who get cancer have likely also consumed a large variety of phytochemicals in their life. In conclusion, the cancer-fighting prowess of phytochemicals has not yet been definitively proved.

Disadvantages of Vegetarian and Vegan Diets

Vegetarians and vegans must always be on the lookout for dietary protein. The protein amounts and quality supplied by plant foods usually does not match the protein of animal foods. It is especially important for vegetarians and vegans to get a broad variety of foods to ensure an adequate variety of dietary amino acids. By knowing how to select complementary proteins, a person can get all the amino acids needed in amounts and proportions correct for human metabolism.

These diets are also sometimes short in vitamin B12, calcium, and vitamin D, which are usually supplied by dairy products.

Vegans have added worries about getting enough iron, zinc, and omega-3 fatty acids. Grains supply good amounts of iron and zinc, but diets high in fiber also bind most of these minerals and make them unavailable for absorption. Omega-3 fatty acids go missing from many diets that exclude seafood.

To make up for some of the potential nutrient deficiencies of vegan diets, follow these tips:

➤ Use a variety of proteins from different legumes, nuts, and soybean products, such as tofu, to assure that the proteins are complementary.

➤ Consider taking a multivitamin to supply vitamin B12, riboflavin, and vitamin D with the addition of the minerals calcium, iron, and zinc. Check with your doctor before taking any multivitamin.

➤ Use iodized salt, especially if abstaining from seafood.

➤ Add some canola or soybean oil, seaweed, flax seeds, microalgae, or walnuts to the diet as a source of omega-3 fatty acids.

➤ Avoid taking in too much fiber.

Macrobiotic Diets

A macrobiotic diet emphasizes whole grains supplemented with vegetables (including sea vegetables), beans, fish, and seafood. Macrobiotic diets exclude meat, eggs, and dairy products and reduce the intake of refined foods, sugar, sodium, and fat.

Macrobiotic diets can be healthy and are believed to be particularly useful in preventing cancer or the reoccurrence of cancers. These diets are nevertheless fairly restrictive so care must be taken to ensure that all required nutrients are either supplied by the diet or taken as supplements.

Nutrition Vocabulary

Micro-algae are edible forms of green algae that provide dietary antioxidants, B vitamins, minerals, and amino acids and other nitrogen sources. Two types have become the most common in dietary supplements: *Spirulina* and *Chlorella*. *Spirulina* is actually not an alga but a bacterium belonging to a group called cyanobacteria. Both cyanobacteria and green algae are similar because they perform photosynthesis and, as such, are Earth's major sources of the oxygen we breathe. Both microbes have been used for centuries as food, often as sun-dried cakes eaten raw or cooked. In Western cultures, micro-algae supplements usually are in capsule form.

Training Diets

Training diets are designed by nutritionists for people preparing for intensive athletic competition or similar endurance activity. Before beginning any training diet, seek advice from a physician to assure you have no injuries or chronic health concerns. Your next concern is the amount of manipulation you intend to do to your normal diet to achieve better athletic performance.

Some training diets adjust a person's normal diet appropriately to meet the added demands of their musculature, circulatory system, and nervous system. Other training diets have evolved into more extreme modifications of a normal balanced diet. These extreme diets may be safe in the short-term but very damaging to health over longer periods.

Special supplements for training have grown into a big business. People spend about $20 billion annually on dietary supplements to give their body an ergogenic advantage. Athletes and wannabes have gobbled up tons of substances such as bee pollen, beef gland extracts, freeze-dried liver flakes, ginseng, gelatin, seaweed, and artichoke hearts, plus a dizzying variety of protein powders to get what they know as the edge.

The U.S. Food and Drug Administration oversees food additives, but supplements are not as strictly controlled as drugs, so many additives in supplements enter the market with little or no scientific testing.

Nutrition Vocabulary

An ergogenic substance is a work-producing substance. The term *ergo* means work and *genic* means production. For example, a glucogenic substance is one that produces glucose.

Ergogenic aids can be a chemical, such as a dietary supplement, or a drug, a psychological effect, or a mechanical object. Many of today's ergogenic supplements have been popularized by word-of-mouth in gyms and in sports clubs, but the scientific evidence of their action remains scant. As long as an ergogenic substance does not harm the body, perhaps its greatest benefit is the psychological boost it gives a person about to undertake a challenging athletic event. The situation known as mind over matter has been valuable time and again in athletic success.

Nutritionists believe that the following approaches to training diets are safe:

➤ Increased calorie intake to meet the increased energy output

➤ Increased shift toward protein foods to help build musculature

➤ Vitamin and mineral supplements for the increased energy metabolism

➤ Extra water intake to support all the increases in metabolic reactions

➤ Sports drinks for hydration and to replace electrolytes lost through perspiration

➤ Energy bars or meal replacement drinks (Ensure Plus or Boost) in short-term use of a few weeks

Some nutritionists also permit the short-term use of the following for giving a boost to athletic performance:

➤ Caffeine

➤ Creatine

➤ Sodium bicarbonate (baking soda) (Baking soda dissolved in water at a ratio of 135 milligrams per pound of body weight and taken one to three hours before competition is believed to help remove excess lactic acid buildup from muscles.)

Supplements to avoid or that have insufficient data on their safety are:

➤ Anabolic steroids

➤ Growth hormone

➤ Glutamine

➤ Branched-chain amino acids

➤ Gamma hydroxybutyrate (GHB)

➤ Beta-Hydroxy beta-methylbutyric acid (HMB)

➤ Erythropoietin (Epogen)

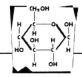

The Chemistry of Nutrition

Creatine is a four-carbon, nitrogen-containing substance sold in crystals to supplement protein drinks. The body's cells readily absorb creatine and quickly combine it with phosphate to make phosphocreatine. The bond linking the phosphate to the creatine molecule is similar to the high-energy bond of ATP. For this reason, phosphocreatine is believed to serve as an added energy source in metabolism.

Phosphocreatine releases its energy only during short bursts of work called anaerobic exercise. Therefore, athletes who need short bursts of energy, such as sprinters and power lifters, may benefit by taking it. They take about 20 grams per day for up to six days before an event and then 2 grams daily on each day of competition. Endurance athletes, such as marathoners and triathletes, would not benefit from creatine supplements.

Other Diet Modifications

Decades of nutrition research have added to our knowledge of how the body's needs shift under certain circumstances. For example, we know that stress, however difficult stress is to define, can interfere with nutrient use. Specific age and health conditions in adults are now addressed by modifying their diet.

Important diet modifications for special life circumstances have been published for pregnancy, the elderly, and for people at high risk for cardiovascular disease.

Pregnancy Diets

Pregnancy diets are adjusted for safe weight gain to nourish the fetus; proper caloric intake to support both the mother and the fetus without excessive weight gain; adequate calcium, folate, and other vitamin and mineral intakes; and adjusted protein, carbohydrate, and lipid intakes.

The following guidelines are starting points for further research on a pregnancy diet:

➤ Caloric intake increased depending on the mother's initial BMI. Allowable weight gain for pregnancy is usually between 15 and 35 pounds for all women of various BMIs.

➤ Protein increased to 25 grams per day.

➤ Carbohydrate increased to 175 grams per day.

➤ Fat intake increased to 20–30 percent of total calories.

➤ B vitamin intake increased to up to 30 percent; up to 45 percent increase for vitamin B6; and up to 50 percent increase for folate.

➤ Iron intake increased to about 27 milligrams per day.

➤ Iodide increased to 220 micrograms per day.

➤ Zinc and calcium monitored carefully to ensure normal intake is met.

Pregnancy diets also reference specific restrictions on alcohol intake and have recommendations for exercise.

Diets for the Elderly

As the U.S. population ages, the term *elderly* changes to mean different ages to different people. Most of us would no longer consider a recently retired person of age sixty-five to be elderly. For this nutrition discussion, an elderly person is a man or woman whose normal activities have decreased so that energy intake can also be decreased.

The elderly need the same balanced diet as a younger adult. Some modifications are appropriate for the elderly, however, such as these:

➤ More frequent, smaller meals to aid digestion

➤ Emphasis on nutrient-dense foods to ensure a balanced diet

➤ Adequate water intake to help all aspects of digestion, elimination, and metabolism

➤ Easy-to-prepare foods for days when you are not feeling well or are tired

➤ New seasonings to replace salt

➤ Continued exercise

Low-salt diets are recommended for the elderly to help control hypertension. Adjustments to remove salt from a diet include easy steps, such as:

➤ Buying low-salt or no-salt versions of canned soups, vegetables, and prepared meals

➤ Avoiding the salt shaker and replacing salt with pepper or other seasonings

➤ Eliminating high-salt snacks such as potato chips, pretzels, and pizza

Fad Diets with Staying Power?

Low-carb diets were once quirky approaches to weight loss. Now restricting carbohydrates is a viable way to control calorie intake. Thus, some diets once described as fads have become more accepted in mainstream nutrition.

The Atkins Diet, South Beach Diet, and the Zone Diet are all based on the understanding that some of the carbons from carbohydrate can end up in fats in your body. The hormone insulin is the determining factor in where the carbons go. Thus, each of these diets restricts carbohydrate intake relative to fat and protein intake to control insulin activity. They all call upon the basic biochemistry of nutrition I discussed in Chapter 21: carbohydrates, proteins, and fats do not get used in sequence by the body, but rather they are used faster or slower depending on your intake and output requirements.

Mediterranean Diet

The Mediterranean diet, also called the Sunshine Diet, may be the latest fad diet with staying power because it is already receiving endorsements from the medical establishment.

A Mediterranean diet consists mainly of vegetables, fruits, nuts, seeds, and whole grains with fats supplied mainly from olive oil. This gives a person a good source of fiber, vitamins, minerals, and unsaturated fatty acids. Seafood supplies most of the protein instead of red meat. This supplies omega-3 fatty acids and reduces the proportion of saturated and trans fats. The overall result is what nutritionists have long called a heart-healthy diet.

The Mediterranean diet is based on the predominant foods of the Italian and Greek coasts along the Mediterranean Sea. The features of this diet are the same as doctors and nutritionists have long recommended for good nutrition, but because it is appealing—think red wine and delicious fruit yogurts—it may be successful in getting many people to eat correctly.

Highlights of the Mediterranean diet are:

➤ Frequent meals with smaller portions

➤ Emphasis on fresh fruits and vegetables, legumes, seeds and nuts, yogurt for the dairy portion, seafood for the protein group, olive oil for fats, and small servings of wine

➤ Emphasis on salmon as a main ingredient of many meals

➤ Emphasis on the vegetables tomato, broccoli, pepper, capers, spinach, eggplant, mushroom, white beans, lentils, and garbanzo beans (chickpeas)

➤ Restrictive toward simple carbohydrates (sugars and starches) but healthy in fiber and complex carbohydrates

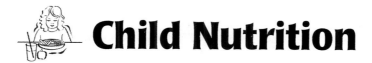

CHAPTER 25

Child Nutrition

In This Chapter

➤ Characteristics of diets for the young

➤ Infant and preschool children nutrition

➤ School-age children and adolescent nutrition

➤ Children's food group requirements

In this chapter you will learn the highlights of nutrition for the growing bodies of infants, toddlers, young children, and adolescents. Logic should tell you that the nutrient needs of a growing youngster will differ from that of an adult or an elderly person. The basics of a balanced diet stay the same, but the demands of bone growth, nerve and muscle development, and rapidly growing tissue make childhood nutrition a separate area study within nutrition.

The habits and behaviors of families also influence the eating habits of a youngster. Some bad eating habits can cause problems later in life. Researchers are learning that the current obesity problem in the United States may have begun for many people very early in their childhood.

This chapter describes the current recommendations for childhood nutrition in various stages of a youngster's growth from infancy to young adulthood.

Hallmarks of a Growing Body

The growing body of any young animal differs from the fully grown adult in a number of key ways. Since the only way a body can grow is to take in plenty of energy and nutrients, nutrition is a critical aspect of growth. Along with emotional nurturing, nutrition is the most important aspect of a newborn's life.

Here are some of the characteristics of growth that are not as important or completely absent in later life:

➤ Cell differentiation and rapid cell replication

➤ Fast growth of long bones so that body length may increase 50 percent in the first year

➤ Increase in the number of adipose cells

➤ Development of brain tissue and growth of nerves

➤ Development of certain sensory preferences, including favorite foods and flavors

Infant Nutrition

There is a reason babies seem only to eat and sleep: they are building new tissue at an extraordinary speed, which takes a lot of work. Work requires lots of nutrients and plenty of rest to recuperate and begin it all anew the next day. Infants have special nutritional needs for a period of life in which they will double in weight the first four to six months, and triple their weight in the first year.

A baby's physician will plan a nutritional schedule for a mother and her baby to meet the energy and nutrient needs of the infant as well as the needs of a mother who is recuperating from pregnancy, returning to a non-pregnancy hormonal balance, and producing milk for a suckling infant. All the while, a mother must keep her energy levels high enough to meet the demands of caring for a new child.

The details of infant nutrition are available in hundreds of resources, beginning with your baby's physician. Here are the highlights of infant nutritional needs:

➤ Calories: From 0 to three months infants need 89 kcal X body weight (in kilograms) + 75. From four to six months infants need 89 kcal X body weight (in kilograms) + 44. From seven to twelve months, infants need 89 kcal X body weight (in kilograms) - 78.

➤ Protein: Requirements are about 9 grams of protein up to six months of age and about 14 grams for older infants (seven to twelve months).

➤ Carbohydrate: Requirements are about 60 grams up to six months of age, and about 95 grams for older infants.

➤ Fat: The infant's requirement is about 30 grams of fat per day with essential fatty acids making up 15 percent of the total fat intake.

➤ Vitamins: Infants should get supplements of vitamin K, D, and B12 under the direction of the baby's physician.

➤ Minerals: Infants usually need supplemental iron, zinc, iodide, and fluoride.

➤ Water: Infants need about 3 cups of water per day. Most of this comes from breast milk or formula. In hot weather, extra water is needed to prevent dehydration, which occurs faster in infants than in adults.

➤ Sleep: Adequate sleep is needed for managing energy metabolism and giving time for the body to distribute and store nutrients and build new cells.

Formula

Formula is a nutrient substitute for breast milk. Most formula manufacturers replace cow's milk or alter it because an infant's digestive tract cannot tolerate large amounts of this milk.

Several commercial preparations of formula are available to provide full nutrition for a period of an infant's life. There are no nutritional advantages or disadvantages between prepared, powdered, or concentrated versions.

Nutrition Morsels

Colostrum is the first fluid secreted by the breast in late pregnancy and in the first two to three days after birth. Colostrum is thicker than subsequent breast milk and contains elevated calories plus high amounts of proteins and substances to boost the baby's immunity. The immune proteins in colostrum are called globulins.

Weaning

At about six months of age, an infant can begin to be weaned from breast milk and bottle feeding. Continued drinking from a bottle bathes teeth in simple carbohydrates that cause dental caries. Drinking from sippy cups reduce the exposure of teeth to the liquid and thus reduces the risk of early childhood caries.

By about ten months, a child is ready to self-feed and drink independently from a cup, although the attempts are often messy!

The transition from a regular milk diet to a regular solid diet can follow these guidelines:

➤ Build gradually from limited variety of foods to a wider variety.

➤ Introduce vegetables and fruits early but beware of adding too much fiber. High-fiber diets safe for adults are not good for infants.

➤ Include some fat. Fat is an essential nutrient at all ages.

➤ Moderate the intake of simple carbohydrates, sugars, and salt can help develop healthy eating habits for later life.

➤ Focus on calcium, iron, and zinc, which can easily be deficient in growing children.

Physicians will advise other guidelines for good infant nutrition. Among these are a list of foods to avoid, such as sugar, honey, small-bite foods that can cause choking, cow's milk (especially fat-free or low-fat), and excessive amounts of fruit juices.

Standard infant feeding recommendations are:

➤ Breastfeeding can continue for six to eight months until breast milk production declines.

➤ Breastfeeding usually calls for vitamin D supplements and possibly added vitamin B12, iron, and fluoride.

➤ Formula for formula-fed infants can be fed for the first year and should be iron fortified.

➤ Iron-fortified cereals can be introduced to all children beginning at six months of age.

➤ The introduction of soft foods can begin at six months and the variety increased gradually.

Nutrition for Young Children

Young children continue to need a balanced nutrient supply in amounts that meet their fast growth. Unfortunately, many preschool children begin to develop eating tendencies that threaten their chances of getting a well-balanced diet. The sometimes strange food preferences of young children are due in part to a high proportion of extra-sensitive taste buds. Other eating behaviors have psychological foundations and can be quite exasperating for parents. Know that as a parent, you may be confronted with these challenges of childhood nutrition:

➤ Picky eaters: Food likes and dislikes change rapidly in children. Parents who are patient and persevere rather than force their child to eat or make deals at mealtime, such as swapping ice cream for carrots, will overcome the period of picky eating.

➤ Rejection of hot foods: It's okay. Heating does not affect the nutrient content of the foods children are likely to eat.

➤ Dislike of vegetables: This is usually balanced by a preference for fruits, which should deliver the needed vitamins, minerals, and carbohydrates.

➤ Disinterest at mealtime: Young children find far more things in their world suitable for exploring than you do at mealtime. An occasional skipped or unfinished meal should not be cause for worry.

➤ Preference for snacking over meals: A child's stomach is small. Frequent small meals may make more sense in the long run than big meals.

A parent's job during this time is to distinguish true eating habits from a child's first forays into exerting independence. Mealtime disagreements should not escalate into full-blown battles. Parents must call upon their skills in psychology, patience, and perseverance—there are those words again—to raise a happy, confident child while also ensuring their child's good nutrition. No easy task!

Nutrition for School Children and Adolescents

In school years, a child's eating habits come under significant influence from peers. Parents have discovered that most of the peer pressure seems to lead away from good nutrition rather than toward it. Despite the best efforts of schools, dieticians, and parents, most children in the United States do not eat enough fresh vegetables, fruit, whole grains, or dairy products. Iron, zinc, and calcium intake are often deficient. Meanwhile, sugary snacks and drinks and salty foods predominate.

I would need another whole book to tackle the problems of school-age children's and adolescents' nutrition. Without that luxury, I include a list of snacks that boost nutrition in children even if they have a sweet tooth or tend to grab chips for lunch instead of chicken salad. Consider these nutrient-dense foods as snacks or supplements to breakfast and lunch:

➤ Calcium snacks: Almonds, cheese on whole wheat crackers, yogurt with granola topping, or bean and cheese burrito

➤ Iron and zinc snacks: Hard-boiled egg, mini-pizza on whole grain muffin, trail mix, tuna salad, whole grain cereal, bean and cheese burrito, whole wheat pasta with vegetables, or peanut butter on apple slices (for zinc only)

➤ Snacks for vitamin C and other antioxidants: Applesauce, dried cranberries, fresh berries, fruit smoothie, fruit salad, or whole wheat pasta with vegetables

➤ Fiber snacks: Popcorn (unbuttered), whole grain cereal, granola, fresh fruit salad, or frozen fruit pieces

Notice that for young adults, it is important to begin increasing the fiber content of their diet. Increased fiber helps control weight gain and aids overall digestion.

Nutrition Morsels

Junk food is any food that delivers empty calories, has high energy density, or is high in fat at the expense of protein and fiber. Fast-food restaurants have unfairly become known as purveyors of junk food, but with careful selection from a fast-food menu you can eat healthy and avoid the pitfalls of junk food.

Many young adults do not, however, make careful selections at lunchtime when they crowd into fast-food restaurants with their friends. They tend to order deep-fried foods instead of salads and fruit cups. Vending machines also offer junk food, sometimes exclusively. School cafeterias have recently made attempts to replace what nutritionists call junk food with foods of lower fat and carbohydrate content and higher fiber. This is a step in the right direction.

Childhood Food Group Requirements

The following are the USDA's recommended levels for a balanced diet for children:

> ➤ Two to three years: 1 cup vegetables, 3 ounces grain equivalents, 2 ounces protein equivalents, 1–1.5 cups fruit, 2 cups dairy

> ➤ Four to eight years: 1.5 cups vegetables, 5 ounces grain equivalents, 4 ounces protein equivalents, 1–1.5 cups fruit, 2.5 cups dairy

> ➤ Nine to thirteen years, girls: 2 cups vegetables, 5 ounces grain equivalents, 5 ounces protein equivalents, 1.5 cups fruit, 3 cups dairy

> ➤ Nine to thirteen years, boys: 2.5 cups vegetables, 6 ounces grain equivalents, 5 ounces protein equivalents, 1.5 cups fruit, 3 cups dairy

> ➤ Fourteen to eighteen years, girls: 2.5 cups vegetables, 6 ounces grain equivalents, 5 ounces protein equivalents, 1.5 cups fruit, 3 cups dairy

> ➤ Fourteen to eighteen years, boys: 3 cups vegetables, 8 ounces grain equivalents, 6.5 ounces protein equivalents, 2 cups fruit, 3 cups dairy

See Chapter 21 for the foods that meet these requirements and the meaning of ounce equivalents.

CHAPTER 26

 # Nutrient Imbalance: Malnutrition

In This Chapter

➤ Types and causes of malnutrition

➤ Main nutrient deficiency diseases

➤ Features of nutrient malabsorption diseases

In this chapter I cover malnutrition. The prefix *mal* refers to any poor or abnormal health condition. We tend to connect malnutrition with nutrient deficiency, but malnutrition can also come from an overabundance of a dietary nutrient that interferes with normal metabolism. Thus scurvy is a malnutrition condition caused by a deficiency of vitamin C. But obesity is also a form of malnutrition because it is caused by an excessive intake of food, leading to poor overall health.

Malnutrition is a worldwide problem that Americans may believe is nonexistent in this country. In industrialized parts of the world, including the United States, malnutrition is caused by overconsumption of foods. Estimates of the percentage of people who are overweight in the United States range from 35 to 50 percent. About 35 percent of the adult U.S. population is obese.

In other parts of the world, malnutrition is commonly caused by undernutrition (long-term inadequate nutrient and calorie intake) rather than overnutrition (overeating).

The Roots of Malnutrition

Undernutrition occurs on every continent except Antarctica. In both the industrialized world and poor countries, the main causes of undernutrition are poverty, chronic illness, alcoholism, and nutrient-restrictive diets. In the poorest parts of the world, people are malnourished mainly due to deficiencies of protein, iron, zinc, and vitamins.

Undernutrition takes two forms. One is the circumstance of being underfed for a long time or throughout a lifetime. Malnourished people get inadequate energy and nutrients to sustain normal metabolism. The other form of undernutrition involves a deficiency of a single nutrient. Often these nutrient deficiency diseases are well defined and studied and can be corrected by returning the missing nutrient to the diet. These diseases are listed later in this chapter.

Overnutrition occurs mainly because of overeating that has been made possible by affluence, simply a restaurant-on-every-corner syndrome. But affluence is not the whole story behind obesity. Certain geographic regions have higher percentages of obesity than others. Furthermore, people at the lower end of the economic spectrum tend to have higher rates of obesity than more affluent people. Overnutrition is a complicated issue affected by interrelated socioeconomic, psychological, and genetic factors.

Another major cause of overnutrition is intoxication by taking an excess of one or a few nutrients. For example, vitamin A toxicity is a form of overnutrition.

The Main Malnutrition Diseases

Malnutrition diseases vary across age groups and according to the nutrients that are out of balance in the diet. Several dozen malnutrition diseases are known. The following examples represent the variety and amount of food groups eaten rather than a single nutrient deficiency in the diet:

> ➤ Loss of subcutaneous fat
> ➤ Skin abnormalities: cracking, dryness, pallor, mouth sores, spongy and bleeding gums
> ➤ Abnormal color and texture of the tongue
> ➤ Poor muscle tone
> ➤ Decreased function in sensory systems
> ➤ Anemia
> ➤ Various inflammations
> ➤ Abnormalities of the cornea and conjunctiva
> ➤ Chest deformity and poor posture

Some of these undefined symptoms of malnutrition are collectively referred to as wasting.

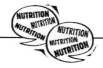

Nutrition Vocabulary

Wasting is any condition of becoming weak, emaciated, and decreased in size due to a disappearance of body protein and fat. In human nutrition, wasting is a general sign of malnutrition, usually undernutrition. In animal nutrition, chronic wasting disease is caused by infection of deer, elk, and moose by infectious proteins called prions. This animal disease is also called transmissible spongiform encephalopathy. The human and animal forms of wasting are unrelated.

Nutrient Deficiency Diseases

The following are the main nutrient deficiency diseases that in impoverished parts of the world tend to accompany undernutrition:

➤ Goiter: Iodide deficiency that causes enlarged thyroid gland. It is common in parts of South America, Africa, and Eastern Europe and can be corrected by adding iodized salt or saltwater fish to the diet.

➤ Anemia: From iron deficiency, although other nutrient deficiencies can lead to anemia. Occurs worldwide and can be corrected by adding a variety of iron-containing foods to the diet: meat, seafood, green vegetables, whole grains, and iron-enriched foods.

➤ Xerophthalmia: Vitamin A deficiency that causes blindness. It is most common in parts of Asia and Africa and can be prevented by adding vitamin A foods to the diet: fortified milk, carrots, sweet potatoes, apricots, cantaloupe, and green leafy vegetables.

➤ Beriberi: Thiamin deficiency causing nerve degeneration, muscle incoordination, and cardiovascular weakness. It occurs in famine-stricken parts of the world and can be prevented by adding meats, seeds, grains, and dried beans to the diet.

➤ Pellagra: A niacin deficiency causing diarrhea, dermatitis, and dementia. It occurs in famine-stricken parts of the world and can be prevented by adding tuna, beef, chicken, whole grains, peanuts, and mushrooms to the diet.

➤ Rickets: A vitamin D deficiency causing poorly calcified and formed bones. It is most common in cultures requiring women and children to cover their bodies, preventing skin exposure to sunlight and can be prevented by adding fortified milk and fish oils to the diet, and being exposed to sunlight.

➤ Scurvy: A vitamin C deficiency that leads to poor wound healing and abnormal bleeding of skin, gums, and internal tissues. It occurs in famine-stricken parts of the world and can be corrected by adding citrus fruits and green vegetables (broccoli) to the diet.

➤ Megaloblastic anemia: A folate deficiency occurring mainly in Africa and Asia. It can be corrected by adding green leafy vegetables, legumes, oranges, and liver to the diet.

➤ Ariboflavinosis: A riboflavin deficiency seen as an inflammation in the mouth and nervous system disorders. It occurs in famine-stricken parts of the world and can be corrected by adding good B vitamin sources such as milk, mushrooms, spinach, liver, and enriched grains to the diet.

Malabsorption

Malabsorption is the inadequate absorption of nutrients from the digestive tract into the bloodstream. It occurs mainly in the small intestine. Many diseases can interfere with nutrient absorption. Diseases affecting the intestinal mucosa, infections, or pancreatic disease that reduces the secretion of digestive enzymes can all lead to nutrient malabsorption.

Two important malabsorption diseases are Crohn's disease and celiac disease. A less common problem in mineral absorption called Wilson's disease is also discussed below.

Crohn's disease

Crohn's disease is an inflammation of the digestive tract that can arise anywhere from the mouth to the anus. The inflammations usually occur in patches and seem to be most common in the last section of the small intestine (ileum) and first section of the large intestine. Crohn's disease is believed to be caused by an overreaction of the body's immune system to its own intestinal lining. In some people with the disease, the cause may be genetic.

In Crohn's disease, the inflammation causes a thickening of the intestinal wall and malabsorption in the affected patches. Absorption of vitamins, minerals, and fats may be most affected, but the peculiarities of the malabsorption vary from person to person.

Symptoms include unexplained weight loss, abdominal pain, fever, fatigue, and persistent diarrhea.

Crohn's disease has no known cure and the dietary treatments vary from person to person. People with the disease should focus on a balanced diet emphasizing nutrient-dense foods.

Several small meals throughout the day may be helpful. Sufferers are also advised to drink plenty of water to aid digestion and replace fluids lost with diarrhea. High-fat, high-fiber, and dairy foods sometimes aggravate Crohn's disease symptoms.

This disease was named for the American gastroenterologist Burrill B. Crohn (pronounced krōn). He was the first to describe this disease in the 1930s.

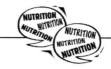

Nutrition Vocabulary

Gastroenterology is a branch of medical science that studies the workings of the stomach and intestines and related organs, such as the esophagus, liver, gallbladder, and pancreas.

Celiac Disease

Celiac disease is caused either by an allergic reaction or a person's own immune system, which has a pronounced reaction to the protein gluten. Gluten occurs in many grains such as wheat, barley, and rye. Some people's sensitivity to gluten is strong enough so that they can be affected by contamination of gluten foods on breadboards and in toasters, even when preparing gluten-free foods.

In celiac disease, the small hairlike projections lining the small intestine become damaged. This reduces the intestine's ability to absorb nutrients. Eventually, a person with celiac disease becomes malnourished even when eating plenty of food and a balanced diet.

Symptoms include unexplained weight loss, abdominal pain, diarrhea or constipation, nausea, and possible vomiting.

Celiac disease has no cure, but people diagnosed with the disease can adhere to a gluten-free diet, which allows time for the intestinal lining to heal. Many gluten-free foods are now available in groceries, and restaurants have made attempts to offer gluten-free dishes. Assuming no contamination has occurred from gluten-containing foods, this diet can return a person to full health and good nutrition.

Wilson's Disease

Wilson's disease is an inherited malabsorption condition in which a person absorbs too much dietary copper. The metal accumulates in organs, eventually shutting down normal function in the liver, brain, spleen, kidneys, and other tissues.

The untreated disease is fatal. Treatment involves a diet that avoids known copper-containing foods (organ meats, shellfish, nuts, dried legumes, whole cereals, and chocolate). Treatment usually also includes an additive to the diet, such as D-penicillamine, which binds copper in the digestive tract and makes it unavailable for absorption.

This disease was named for the American-born, British-educated internist Samuel A. K. Wilson who first described the disease in the early 1900s. A bit of an eccentric, Wilson preferred that his colleagues call the disease Kinnier Wilson's disease because he preferred Kinnier as his surname.

Protein-Energy Malnutrition

This type of malnutrition is from a deficiency of protein and energy at the same time. Protein-energy malnutrition is most common in children younger than five years, people with chronic illness, critically ill patients, and in famine.

In protein-energy malnutrition, the body begins breaking down muscle proteins to use amino acid for energy. Muscle tone decreases and eventually the heart weakens. The two most serious protein-energy malnutrition diseases seen in impoverished parts of the world are kwashiorkor and marasmus.

Kwashiorkor and Marasmus

Kwashiorkor is a disease of malnourished and protein-deficient children. The signs begin to develop soon after weaning and include lethargy, apathy, failure to grow, mental deficiency, dermatitis, and an enlarged liver.

Many ailments accompany children with kwashiorkor, but treatment can reverse some symptoms. A gradual introduction of a protein-sufficient balanced diet must be done with a physician's supervision.

Marasmus is a general emaciation and loss of subcutaneous fat due to protein-energy deficiency. Symptoms include hair loss, decreased muscle mass, and a sunken face. In long-term cases, individuals have heads that appear too large for their emaciated bodies.

These two diseases are similar with similar devastating effects on body metabolism. The main distinction between the two is noticeable edema (fluid retention) in kwashiorkor victims, seen as an extended abdomen, and the lack of edema in marasmus victims.

Both diseases are seen worldwide in the poorest regions affected by chronic hunger. They also occur, but more rarely, in North America.

CHAPTER 27

Nutrition-Related Diseases

In This Chapter

➤ Descriptions of common food- or nutrition-related diseases

➤ Distinguishing food allergies, sensitivities, and intolerances

---

In this chapter you learn more about diseases related to nutrition. I begin with the most common food illness of all: foodborne infections, which range from minor inconvenience to life-threatening events. Sooner or later everyone gets a foodborne infection.

This chapter also covers the main nutrition-related diseases that are common in North America. It is likely that you or someone you know will suffer from one of these illnesses. Fortunately, these diseases receive a considerable amount of study by nutrition researchers and the medical community. Therefore, preventions and treatments are usually well known.

Foodborne Illness

You might refer to this group of illnesses as food poisoning. Foodborne illness is an infection caused by microbes that have contaminated food. The common perpetrators are bacteria, viruses, molds, and protozoa. In some parts of the world, parasites (worms, larvae, insects, etc.) also present a problem.

Foodborne illnesses are of two main types: those caused by the microbe and those caused by a toxin (a biological poison) secreted by the microbe, called an intoxication.

Foodborne illnesses are among the most common illnesses seen each year. In most cases, these microbes are ingested from contaminated food or contaminated water. They are becoming more common because of our increasingly centralized method of processing foods.

Microbes that cause foodborne illnesses are invisible, and often the only clue of illness comes from telltale signs of "something I ate," which are nausea, vomiting, headache, possible fever and chills, weakness, abdominal cramping, and diarrhea. Thousands of cases occur every year in the United States, but undoubtedly many additional cases are never reported to a doctor. Several hundred deaths occur each year due to foodborne illness. The majority of foodborne illnesses are caused by these microbes:

➤ Bacteria: *Staphylococcus aureus, Bacillus cereus, Clostridium botulinum, Clostridium perfringens, Escherichia coli (E. coli), Listeria monocytogenes, Campylobacter jejuni, Vibrio cholerae, Salmonella, Shigella*, and *Yersinia*

➤ Viruses: Hepatitis A, enterovirus, norovirus, and rotavirus.

➤ Molds: *Claviceps purpurea, Aspergillus, Penicillium*, and *Fusarium*

➤ Protozoa: *Cryptosporidium*

Of these microbes, the following also produce toxins that sometimes do more damage in the body than the live microbe:

➤ Bacteria: *Staphylococcus, E. coli, Clostridium, Shigella*

➤ Molds: *Claviceps, Aspergillus, Penicillium*, and *Fusarium*

Microbial toxins are dangerous in foods because even after cooking food to kill the microbes, the toxin remains in the food and is able to cause illness.

Severe foodborne illness can interfere with nutrition due to nutrient, energy, and water loss during diarrhea. Loss of appetite, nausea, and vomiting also disrupt a normal diet.

Food Allergies

Food allergies are also very common and may be increasing in the U.S. population. Each year, food allergies cause about 30,000 visits to emergency rooms and 200 deaths.

A food allergy is a dramatic reaction by the body to a substance it perceives as foreign. This allergy-causing foreign substance is called an allergen and is usually made of protein.

Nutritionists separate food allergies into three general groups based on their symptoms. An allergy-sufferer may not get all these symptoms with each episode but will probably experience at least two or three:

1. Classic allergies: Itching, reddened skin, swelling, asthma, runny nose, and choking

2. General allergies: Headache, skin rashes, tension, fatigue, tremors, and psychological reactions

3. Gastrointestinal allergies: Nausea, vomiting, diarrhea, gas, bloating, abdominal pain, constipation, and indigestion

Nutrition Vocabulary

Some confusion invariably arises with discussions of allergens, antigens, antibodies, and allergies. An allergen is a protein particle foreign to the body that may cause the body to react to it using the immune system. The first reaction to a new allergen may be mild, but subsequent exposures are often more intense. We know these intense reactions to allergens as an allergic response.

An antigen is a foreign protein that stimulates the immune system to produce antibodies. Antibodies are proteins made by the body's immune system to destroy specific antigens.

All allergens are antigens, but not all antigens are allergens.

Food allergies span a wide range in severity from person to person. Your physiology accounts for much of the symptoms you'll experience with a food allergy. These symptoms may last a few seconds to days. The type of allergen and its dose will certainly impact the severity of the symptoms.

Anaphylactic Shock

A general whole-body and sudden reaction to an allergen is called anaphylactic shock, or anaphylaxis. Within minutes of exposure to an offending allergen, anaphylactic shock causes blood pressure to plummet and can drastically interfere with the respiratory and digestive systems. These whole-body reactions can be fatal if treatment is not administered quickly. Treatment usually involves giving the sufferer antihistamines or epinephrine.

These are the symptoms of severe anaphylactic shock:

➤ Wheezing and extreme difficulty breathing

➤ Confusion, dizziness, and lightheadedness

➤ Rapid swelling over the body

➤ Hives, which are raised, swollen, and very itchy areas on the skin

➤ Blue coloration to the skin

➤ Nausea, vomiting, and diarrhea

Some milder cases of anaphylactic shock can occur and are not life-threatening. Severe hay fever, hives without the other more serious symptoms of anaphylaxis, and some gastrointestinal reactions to foods fall into this category.

Any protein food can cause anaphylactic shock, depending on a person's sensitivity to it, but the main causes are:

➤ Peanuts

➤ Tree nuts (walnuts, almonds, pecans, etc.)

➤ Shellfish

➤ Milk protein (casein)

➤ Egg protein (albumin)

➤ Soybeans

➤ Wheat

➤ Some fish

Some foods contain ingredients made from fish and they too can cause a sudden allergic response. People who know they have an allergic sensitivity to fish should avoid eating Worchester sauce, gelatin, and some omega-3 fatty acid supplements.

Food Sensitivities

A food sensitivity is any reaction similar to the ones listed above for anaphylactic shock, but milder overall. Food sensitivities show up as slight itching of the skin or redness or both.

Food Intolerances

A food intolerance is not an allergic reaction to food, but people often lump intolerances together with food allergies. Food intolerances are mild to severe reactions by the body to a component in a certain food, but the reaction does not involve the immune system. The best example of a food intolerance is lactose intolerance. A person who is lactose intolerant lacks sufficient amounts of the enzyme lactase so cannot digest the sugar lactose in milk and some other dairy products. The undigested sugar becomes food for the large population of bacteria in the intestines. A burst of bacterial growth, happily chomping away on the lactose, causes painful abdominal gas, cramping, and diarrhea.

Other food intolerances can come from specific ingredients in fresh fruits or vegetables, food additives (coloring, preservatives, monosodium glutamate), microbial toxins, or other residual substances from food production such as antibiotics or hormones in meat. Intolerance to the protein gluten, found in wheat and rye, causes a variety of discomforts in sensitive people. A rare but more serious intolerance to gluten, called celiac disease, can damage the cells lining the intestines.

Gas, Heartburn, and Acid Indigestion

These three maladies were for a long time grouped together as the unfortunate outcomes of overeating or eating the "wrong foods." Today, physicians try to determine the exact symptoms you may be experiencing from eating specific foods to find the root cause. They are increasingly finding the cause to be gastroesophageal reflux disease (GERD) or a milder condition simply called gastroesophageal reflux (GER).

Both illnesses are caused by an incomplete closing of the sphincter muscle that shuts the door between the esophagus and your stomach. The faulty closure allows some of the very acidic gastric juices from the stomach to move back up (reflux) the digestive tract into the esophagus. The acids burn the esophageal lining, causing pain. Persistent reflux and burning (GERD) can cause damage to the esophagus.

Some foods may increase GER for some people. The best treatment, of course, is to avoid these foods once you are sure they cause the problem. Your physician may also advise you do the following, if appropriate, to lessen GER's effects:

> ➤ Lose weight

> ➤ Stop smoking

> ➤ Eat smaller, more frequent meals

> ➤ Avoid lying down within three hours after a meal

> ➤ At night, arrange pillows or the bed's headboard so that your head is raised 6–8 inches above your chest.

Some over-the-counter antacids or prescription drugs alleviate GER's symptoms, but they seldom cure the problem permanently.

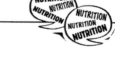

Nutrition Vocabulary

Diagnosing an illness caused by food requires you and your physician to review your signs and symptoms. What is the difference between these two medical terms? A *sign* is a concrete piece of evidence your physician uses to diagnose illness. For example, heart rate, blood cholesterol levels, and yellow skin or jaundice are signs. A *symptom* is a subjective piece of evidence that you, the patient, describe to your doctor. Symptoms include, "I feel lousy today, Doc." Other symptoms are abdominal pain, itchiness, headache, and overall weakness. In other words, a doctor measures signs and you describe symptoms.

Gallstones

Gallstones are pebble-like balls that develop in the gallbladder. They can form when the liver, which is connected to the gallbladder, accumulates either too much cholesterol or too many natural body pigments, and then these substances crystallize if not enough liquid is present. These pebbles might also lodge in the bile ducts, the canals that drain material from the liver to the gallbladder.

Cholesterol gallstones are more common than pigment gallstones. This may not matter much to you if you're suffering from either type. Gallstones cause painful inflammation wherever they lodge. The pain usually occurs in the upper abdomen, in the back between the shoulder blades, or under the right shoulder. Other symptoms are nausea and vomiting, reddish stools, yellowing of the skin (jaundice), and low-grade fever.

High-fat and high-cholesterol diets that are also low in fiber are the main dietary causes of gallstones. They also may be inherited, and women are twice as likely to get gallstones as men, suggesting a hormonal influence. People over sixty years old are also at higher risk for gallstones than those younger.

Gallstones are usually treated only through diet adjustment, such as cutting back on dietary fat and cholesterol. In severe cases, a patient might have the gallbladder removed in a surgical procedure called a cholecystectomy.

Irritable Bowel Syndrome

When you see the word *syndrome* you know the condition has many forms and possibly many causes. A syndrome is a group of symptoms, signs, lab test results, and other abnormalities in one's physiology that add up to a disease.

Irritable bowel syndrome (IBS) is a condition characterized by gas, constipation or diarrhea, frequent bloating, and possible mucus in the stools. These complaints are among the most common reasons people see their physician, yet IBS remains difficult to diagnose and difficult to treat. In severe cases of IBS, a patient might develop fever, lose weight, and have bleeding in the intestines. (Black stools are a sign of intestinal bleeding.)

Your doctor may adjust your diet to alleviate the worst symptoms of IBS. This usually starts by eliminating gas-inducing foods such as dairy products. You may need to increase your fiber to speed the movement of intestinal contents or decrease fiber to cut down on intestinal irritation. Drinking more water almost always helps reduce IBS's symptoms as does increased exercise.

Ulcers

An ulcer is an inflammation of the skin or the mucosa in a concentrated spot. Most people think of gastric ulcers, which are inflammations of the mucosa lining the inside of the stomach. This lining protects the stomach wall from the acidic and very caustic gastric juices in the stomach contents. When an ulcer forms, the acids can burn into your stomach wall, causing pain and bleeding.

Peptic Ulcers

Peptic ulcers are ulcers that occur anywhere from the lower esophagus to the distal end (farthest from the mouth) of the small intestine. For decades, physicians could not find the cause of this common ailment—about 10 percent of people get peptic ulcers. For a long time the cause was chalked up to stress or eating spicy foods.

We now know some of the real causes of peptic ulcers. The two main culprits are the bacteria called *Helicobacter pylori* and nonsteroidal anti-inflammatory drugs (NSAIDs). Either one of these factors can damage the stomach's mucosa and initiate the formation of an ulcer.

The symptoms of peptic ulcers are:

➤ Stomach pain, especially at night

➤ Nausea and/or vomiting

➤ Heartburn (reflux)

➤ Weight loss

Physicians will test your blood for antibodies against *Helicobacter pylori*. If the antibodies are present, this means you have the microbe in your stomach and may be causing the ulcers. A treatment with antibiotics will eliminate the bacteria and possibly solve the ulcer problem too.

If you have been taking NSAIDs for many months and have no signs of the bacteria, then the drugs are probably causing your ulcers. Stopping NSAID use is the first step to recovery. If you need NSAIDS for pain control associated with other health problems, consider doing the following:

➤ Lower the dose

➤ Take the drug only with meals

➤ Stop smoking and/or lower alcohol consumption, which both aggravate the ulcers

Nutrition Vocabulary

Nonsteroidal anti-inflammatory drugs (NSAIDs) are common treatments for chronic (long-term) and acute (sudden, extreme) pain, fever, and inflammation. The most common NSAIDs are aspirin, ibuprofen, naproxen, and ketoprofen.

Pancreatitis

Pancreatitis is an inflammation of the pancreas; the term *itis* always means inflammation. The pancreas is an organ that works with the small intestines to help digestion by secreting into the small intestine an array of enzymes to break down food.

Pancreatitis may take a sudden form (acute pancreatitis) or be more long-lasting, leading to permanent damage of the organ (chronic pancreatitis). This disease may also affect certain parts of the pancreas or only the pancreatic duct, which leads to the duodenum of the small intestine. Any of these inflammations will disrupt the normal flow of enzymes (amylase, lipase, and protease) that play a major role in digestion.

The symptoms of acute pancreatitis, listed below, are often easier to recognize than the chronic form:

➤ Swelling and tenderness of the abdomen

➤ Nausea and vomiting

➤ Fever

➤ Rapid pulse (this is a sign rather than a symptom)

Obviously, your ability to digest a balanced diet will be affected by pancreatitis.

Acute pancreatitis often requires a hospital stay. Intravenous fluids and electrolytes help the symptoms disappear and relieve the inflammation.

CHAPTER 28

How to Read Food Labels

In This Chapter

➤ Food label requirements and items

➤ Information you get from the Nutrition Facts label

➤ The purpose of food additives

In this chapter you take on the fun task of reading food labels. Fortunately, the FDA requires all food manufacturers to label all packaged foods with certain information. If you know what to look for within the food's information label, you can work toward a more balanced diet. This means limiting fat and carbohydrates, which most of us eat in excess, reducing saturated and trans fats, raising fiber intake, and getting the vitamins and minerals that tend to be deficient in our Western diets.

Food Label Requirements

The FDA oversees regulations regarding food labels, called Nutrition Facts, including the information that must appear on this label. In addition to where this label must be placed on a food package, the FDA also enforces requirements for the food's name, logo, and any claims the manufacturer makes about the food. For example, if you see a juice can that claims, "Cures baldness," you should be very suspicious. Most food manufacturers are too savvy to make that mistake, but they might try to push the borders of good sense by making claims in the following areas:

> ➤ A good source of [insert nutrient here]

> ➤ A source of antioxidants

> ➤ A good source of fiber

> ➤ All natural

Manufacturers are also not allowed to make health claims about their foods. Foods cannot cure cancer or any other disease other than a specific nutrient deficiency disease. The FDA tries to catch as many of these false claims before a product reaches consumers, but consumers must be on the lookout for suspicious products too. Some food claims walk the fine line of being legal in FDA's eyes, but are still a bit misleading about the true benefits their product delivers.

Package Label

Food packages must contain the following information:

> ➤ Product name in specific font sizes

> ➤ Manufacturer's name and full address

> ➤ Amount of product in the package

> ➤ List of ingredients

> ➤ A use by date or other indication about the food's shelf life

A food package must also have a clearly identified front, which the FDA calls the principal display panel (PDP). Also, pictures or certain intervening messages ("Tastes great!") cannot distract from the nutritional information that appears on the side or opposite the PDP.

Nutrition Facts Label

Only fresh fruits and vegetables, meats, fish, and poultry do not have to include the Nutrition Facts.

The Nutrition Facts always provide you with the serving size and the number of servings in the container. Most people who try to lose weight may select the right foods but forget about serving size. All the nutritional information on the rest of the label relates to one serving size, so check this first. Sadly, many people eat two, three, or more servings of many packaged foods with each meal. The label always prefaces its nutritional information with qualifying "Amount per Serving."

By looking at any food in your pantry, you can see what information the FDA requires. All foods follow the same format. Let's review to be sure you understand all the information the Nutrition Facts deliver:

➤ The values for calories and calories from fat are in kcal. The calories from fat tell you how fatty this food is. For example, butter has 100 calories and 100 calories from fat printed on its label. A low-fat food contains a much lower proportion of calories from fat. Strive to keep the calories from fat less than total calories. You'll need to do some quick math. If a serving of soup carries 15 calories from fat and 90 total calories, the percent of calories from fat is (15 ÷ 90) x 100 = 16.67 percent.

➤ The next three lines, total fat, saturated fat, and trans fat, tell you the exact amounts in grams (g) of fat in the food and the amounts of the two types you should try to reduce: saturated fat and trans fat. Most foods contain some fat, but try to keep the grams of saturated and trans fats as close to zero as possible.

➤ Cholesterol and sodium content appear on the next two lines. These should also be minimized. Cholesterol in all meals should add up to no more than 300 milligrams per day. Sodium totals should never go over 2,500 milligrams or 2.5 grams per day.

➤ The next three lines show you the food's total carbohydrates, dietary fiber, and sugars in grams. These three lines have different meanings depending on your general health, your need to lose or gain weight, and your age. Normal healthy adults try to eat carbohydrates in moderation, increase their fiber, and decrease their sugar intake. The food label does not tell you which direction you are trying to go for each of these nutrients, but it does provide some guidance by giving you the daily value percentage in a column to the right of the entries from total fat through dietary fiber.

➤ Daily value is a general value based on a 2,000 kcal diet. If you need much more or much less than 2,000 kcal per day, the daily value percentage doesn't help you. For everyone else it gives an idea of whether a food is providing a big slug of the specific nutrient or only a tiny dribble. Most people want to lower their intake of saturated fat, trans fat, cholesterol, sodium, and sugar. Conversely, most people want to increase their fiber intake.

➤ No daily value is given for sugars and protein. This is because an exact recommendation for dietary sugar has never been proposed and because protein content is less important than protein quality. It's too expensive for food companies to analyze the protein quality of their products. In general, try to minimize your sugar intake and eat enough protein so that it totals 10–15 percent of your total energy intake. (See the recommendations below.)

➤ Vitamin A, vitamin C, calcium, and iron listed on the line below protein are shown as percentages of the daily recommended value. Higher numbers tell you that this food does a good job toward meeting your daily requirements. Lower numbers mean that this food isn't helping much and you still need to eat a good source of A, C, calcium, and/or iron.

➤ Many Nutrition Facts labels add a footnote giving you additional information on select nutrients based on a 2,000 kcal diet compared with a 2,500 kcal diet. The footnote focuses on five nutrients that are of special concern to many people: total fat, saturated fat, cholesterol, sodium, and total carbohydrates.

➤ The final required entry is the food product's ingredients listed in order from the ingredient present in the highest amount (by weight) to the lowest amount.

The FDA gives food manufacturers a bit of leeway on what they can put on the Nutrition Facts label. Candy and soft drinks can omit some of the above nutrients and other manufacturers list more nutrients than are required.

Is This a Processed Food?

If it's in a box, bottle, can, or bag, it's a processed food. Any type of handling of a food that gets it from the farm to your table is a form of processing. Fresh vegetables and fruits get minimal processing. They might go through only the following steps:

1. Picking or harvesting

2. Sorting (removing stems, leaves, roots, and rotten pieces or pieces that are too small or immature)

3. Rinsing

4. Boxing, bagging, or canning

After these simple steps, the fresh produce is loaded onto a truck. It then goes to a distribution warehouse, where it stays for a short time (less than twenty-four hours) or a long time (up to two weeks). Some vegetables and fruits go into cold storage for months. Assuming the fresh produce has stopped for only about twenty-four hours, it continues in different trucks to grocery stores or restaurants. Only produce sold at farmers markets come straight from the farm to the consumer. (A few very conscientious restaurant chefs demand that their produce be delivered straight from the farm, but this is rare.)

The fresh produce that does not follow this fairly straightforward route goes to food manufacturing plants. At these plants, the food is handled in a manner that reduces dirt and contamination while preserving as many nutrients as possible. But let's face it, every minute of delay between the farm and you causes some nutrients to go away. The more processing involved, the more nutrients a food is likely to lose. Here are some (but not every) steps that make up our current food-processing extravaganza:

➤ More rinsing and sorting

➤ Peeling

➤ Chopping, dicing, slicing, etc.

➤ Heating or cooking

➤ Mashing, crushing, pureeing, blending, etc.

➤ Mixing with other ingredients, including other foods but also thickeners, emulsifiers, and other texture stabilizers

➤ Adding preservatives, coloring, and flavor enhancers

➤ Freezing, freeze-drying, vacuum-packing, heat-sterilizing, or irradiating

➤ Boxing, bottling, canning, or bagging

➤ Crating and storing

➤ Distributing

By the time you get a food that has made it through processing and distribution, it may seem a miracle you recognize it at all. Today's food industry gets slammed in books, articles, and TV shows on the machinations through which it puts our food. But consider this: we are the most well-fed nation on Earth, with nutrient deficiencies being extremely rare, and almost all children above the poverty line going to school with full stomachs. This is not true for most other parts of the world. Our nutritional problems in the United States come from too much of a good thing: overnutrition. Our processed foods often carry high amounts of fat, saturated and trans fat, nonfood additives, and too much sugar or salt.

I don't think processed foods are signaling the end of civilization as some would have you believe. I do, however, believe that processed foods must fit into the diet the same way you assemble all other food groups, that is, in balance. No one should eat a diet made exclusively of highly processed foods, meaning frozen prepared meals and canned foods. Everyone should do their best to include fresh vegetables and fruits in their balanced diet, focus on minimally processed foods, and eat highly processed foods sparingly. Knowing this, perhaps you can now enjoy that can of Spaghetti-O's!

Meat Processing

Humans are omnivores: we eat both animal foods and plant foods to arrive at balanced nutrition. But we cook most of our animal foods because cooking meat helps us digest meat proteins.

Fresh meats receive extensive processing before you take them home and cook them. Lots of people refuse to think about the process of getting a living animal from the farm to a food that rests between two buns. If you wish to skip this section, you may.

Meat processing involves the following steps:

1. Trucking from pasture to feedlot

2. Fattening at the feedlot

3. Slaughtering

4. Dressing (removing the hide)

5. Rendering (removing fat, bones, hair, feathers, and other nonfood pieces)

6. Cutting

7. Salting or curing (ham, bacon, sausage meats, etc.)

8. Packaging

The cutting step is when the meatpacker prepares large cuts of meat from an animal carcass for a retail butcher. A butcher then cuts up the large pieces to pieces desired by consumers: roasts, briskets, ribs, steaks, breasts, legs, wings, etc.

Meat processing differs from produce processing in one major way: few nutrients are lost in meat processing. Fresh cuts of meat remain good sources of protein, B vitamins, and some minerals.

Find the Preservatives

The real fun begins when you inspect the ingredients list and see a lot of big names that don't appear in cookbooks. These are all food additives.

Food preservatives are chemicals added to food to extend its shelf life. Preservatives inhibit the growth of microbes and minimize the effects of oxygen or metals on the food's flavor and color. Many preservatives are themselves food, so we know they are safe. These preservatives appear on a government list with the catchy title of Generally Recognized as Safe (GRAS). Salt and sugar (honey, invert sugar, corn syrup, etc.) usually help preserve foods. Since we like the taste of salt and sugar, food manufacturers are more than happy to dump them in.

Preservatives and other additives should be used to maintain or improve the quality of the food, which reduces food waste and minimizes foodborne infection. These additives should not be used for deceiving the consumer, covering up poor processing methods, or making unsafe foods appear to be safe.

Other common preservatives are:

> ➤ Ascorbic acid (vitamin C)

> ➤ Benzoic acid, sodium benzoate, and potassium benzoate

➤ Parabens (parahydroxy esters of benzoic acid or parahydroxybenzoic acid)

➤ Acids: Acetic, citric, and sorbic

➤ Calcium propionate

➤ Calcium sorbate, potassium sorbate, and sodium sorbate

➤ Nitrates and nitrites

Most of these preservatives are added into the food product, but sometimes they are merely applied to the wrapping.

Nutrition Morsels

The GRAS list was developed in 1958 so that the food industry would not be required to do extensive safety testing on food additives that people had already been safely eating for decades. The FDA makes this list public. If any item on the GRAS list should be shown to be unhealthy, the FDA has the responsibility of removing it from the list. GRAS list ingredients are used in cosmetics, drugs, plastics, inks, paints, and textiles as well as in foods.

Find All the Other Additives

A food's texture, color, flavor, and general quality, called mouth feel, all influence its appeal to a consumer. Consumers furthermore expect their foods to look and behave certain ways. It seems perfectly acceptable for a bottle of oil and vinegar salad dressing to separate into two phases on a store shelf. People don't mind mixing it before using it. If a jar of mayonnaise similarly separated into its oily, watery, eggy, and other parts, well . . .

Food manufactures put in additives to increase a food's appeal without affecting its nutritional quality:

➤ Color additives: Tartrazine, usually described as FD&C yellow number X.

➤ Flavor additives: Citric acid, calcium lactate, sodium hydroxide, acetic acid, sugar, and salt

➤ Flavor enhancers: Salt and monosodium glutamate (MSG)

➤ Antioxidants: butylated hydroxyanisole (BHA), butylated hydroxytoluene (BHT), α-tocopherol (vitamin E), ascorbic acid, and various sulfites

➤ Emulsifiers: Monoglycerides and lecithin

➤ Humectants (retain moisture): Glycerol, propylene glycol, and sorbitol

➤ Leavening agents: Yeast, baking powder, and baking soda

➤ Curing agents: Salt, nitrates, and nitrites

➤ Maturing agents (conditions flour in baked goods): Bromates, peroxides, and ammonium chloride

The antioxidants used as food additives are not for the supposed health benefits ascribed to these chemicals. Instead, antioxidants work here to inhibit rancidity and prevent chemical reactions in the food that change its color or its safety.

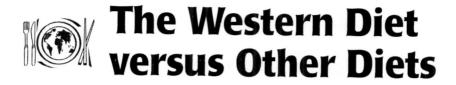 The Western Diet versus Other Diets

In this chapter I take a moment to evaluate what we sometimes call the Western diet. This meat-and-potatoes diet has been blamed for many of the health problems seen in the United States and Europe and for the ongoing issue of overnutrition.

Many people have resisted the trend toward processed, some say overprocessed, foods and have turned to more natural ways of growing and preparing food. We now have organic foods, fair trade foods, dolphin-safe foods, cruelty-free, café-free, rainforest-friendly, and so on. A new food movement has also invented slow food as a not-so-subtle answer to fast food. Do all or any of these specialty foods bring you better nutrition? Do they save the planet or lower our carbon footprint?

This chapter may not answer all those questions, but it will cover the nutritional aspects of foods that make environmental claims. I begin by reviewing the meaning of the Western diet compared with an Eastern diet. I then tackle the sometimes confusing subject of organic foods. Finally, this chapter describes the dizzying variety of environmental labels that show up on foods.

The Main Differences between Western and Other Diets

The Western diet has been tweaked lately to increase fresh vegetables and fruit, but it has always traditionally revolved around meat and potatoes with salad, vegetables, and bread playing supporting roles. Fish, usually deep fried, make rare cameo appearances.

Western diets are high in fat, which is not always bad. Unfortunately, because the Western diet is based on animal sources of protein, the saturated and trans fats and cholesterol can run high. Carbohydrates, including sugar, and salt are usually in excess, and fiber is usually too low. Western diets often include a large portion of meals from fast-food restaurants and pizza parlors. Snacks consist of sweets and salty things that are also often high in fat.

Today's tweaks to the Western diet have added layers of nutritional revelations, but these modifications may not always add up to a balanced diet. We now take lots of supplements, vitamin E, vitamin C, multivitamins, assorted minerals previously known only to ore miners, and antioxidants, by the handful. Do these additions balance the Western diet? Do they reduce the health risks inherent in the Western diet?

Cardiovascular disease, diabetes, food allergies, obesity, hypertension, and other health problems are increasing. Although many factors combine to shift a population's average health, the Western diet has been blamed often.

Nutrition Morsels

If we know all about the Western diet's faults, is there an Eastern diet and does it reverse all the mistakes made by people eating a Western diet?

Eastern diets are associated with the foods of the Far East and Middle East. These diets are often vegetarian but do not require all avoidance of animal foods. They are higher in whole grains, fresh vegetables, fish, and poultry than many Western diets. Although Eastern diets are not perfect—they are often high in simple carbohydrates—they are associated with much lower rates of the heart and weight problems seen with Western diets.

Dietary Supplements

A pill may seem to be an easier way to correct flaws in your diet when compared to watching your intake, focusing on fresh fruits and vegetables, increasing fiber, and exercising. The

FDA does not regulate dietary supplements as strictly as it regulates drugs or even food additives, such as colorings. As a result, dietary supplements may not always be as effective in improving your nutrition as they claim.

The FDA requires that a dietary supplement's package contain a Supplement Facts label. This label is not as information-packed as a food's required Nutrition Facts label. Furthermore, the FDA adds a disclaimer so that if this product doesn't deliver all it claims, the agency bears no responsibility. The disclaimer says, "These statements have not been evaluated by the Food and Drug Administration. This product is not intended to diagnose, treat, cure or prevent any disease."

The information on the Supplement Facts label is:

➤ Serving size and servings per container

➤ Active ingredients listed as amount per serving

➤ Percentage of daily value, usually reported as "Not established"

➤ List of other ingredients

➤ Directions or suggested use

Here are some of the precautions to consider when taking dietary supplements:

➤ They receive minimal testing for effectiveness and safety.

➤ They might contain nutrients in dangerously high amounts.

➤ They often make nutrition and/or health claims that seem too good to be true (because they are).

➤ Claims are often based on few studies, incomplete studies, or very complex studies reduced to simplistic conclusions.

➤ They often hype the popular chemical of the day, such as antioxidants, which have never been proven to be useful in supplement form.

Nutrients in Food Processing and Distribution

Few people would doubt that the more a food is processed, the more the nutrients are likely to disappear. Heating, cooking in water, and storage can lower the nutrient content of many foods. This is one reason why food manufacturers add nutrients back to the food before selling it. Food processing also makes some foods more palatable, easier to digest, and more appealing.

Cooking brings some advantages and disadvantages:

➤ Heating melts fat, causing it to run out of the food and thus lowers your fat intake. Raw foods retain more water-soluble vitamins and minerals than food cooked in water, but the nutrients may be trapped in fiber and unavailable.

➤ Heating breaks down complex carbohydrates to make them more available for digestion and absorption.

➤ Heating makes meat proteins digestible and kills potentially dangerous microbes.

➤ Cooking in water causes water-soluble vitamins to wash away. Steaming retains more of the vitamins than boiling.

Slow Food

Slow food is a philosophy and a environmental/political movement as much as it is an aspect of nutrition. The slow food movement promotes locally grown foods to decrease on the fuels used for transporting traditionally processed foods. Slow foods also focus on fresh vegetables and fruits, minimal processing, and the avoidance of food additives and growth promoters. As with organic food fans, slow food proponents prefer that foods are grown without herbicides, fungicides, or pesticides.

The FDA has no designation or regulations for slow food.

Nutrition Vocabulary

Herbicides, fungicides, and pesticides are three types of chemicals that help crops grow better in fields. Herbicides kill weeds that can crowd food crops and take the crops' water, soil, and sunlight. Fungicides kill molds, which are a type of fungus. Pesticides kill animal pests. This usually means insects (insecticides) and their larvae (larvicides) but can also include poisons that kill vermin, such as rats, mice, and gophers.

Organic Food

To a nutritionist with a background in chemistry, all food is organic. Organic compounds are any chemical that contains carbon. All foods contain carbon and all nutrients other than minerals and water also contain carbon. The term *organic* has nonetheless been adapted in nutrition to mean a food that is produced without any chemical additives. Organic food manufacturers exclude all additives used to promote a food's growth, preserve it, or enhance it.

The USDA oversees the regulations for accepting farms as organic farms and their products as organic food. The USDA allows three designations for organically produced food:

1. The phrase *100 percent organic* means 100 percent of the food's ingredients are organic and were raised in organic conditions.

2. *Organic* means that 95 percent or more of the ingredients are organic as described above.

3. *Made with organic* means that at least 70 percent of the ingredients are organic as described above.

The USDA allows the first two categories of organic foods to display a label on the packaging that states USDA Organic.

Organic Food Claims

Does organic food automatically mean more nutritious food? Not necessarily. A carrot is a carrot. The nutrients in an organic carrot are exactly the same as those in a nonorganic carrot. In fact, in some instances, organic foods are of less value nutritionally than nonorganic versions. Consider the pluses and minuses of organic foods:

➤ Organic foods lack chemicals, so they don't have the health effects these substances may cause in the body.

➤ Organic foods tend to be harvested and shipped in smaller batches, which potentially reduces the nutrient losses that occur with mass production.

➤ Organic foods are allowed to grow in a natural growing season rather than in artificial conditions, which may help nutrient content and flavor or have no effect.

➤ Chemically treated foods have a longer shelf life, thus making the food's nutrients available longer.

➤ Chemically treated foods can grow outside of the natural growing season. This makes fresh fruits and vegetables available to us for a longer part of the year.

➤ Chemically treated produce tends to hold up better during transport than organic fruits and vegetables. This reduces food losses and makes more nutrients available to consumers.

Nutrition Vocabulary

Shelf life is the amount of time a food can be stored before it is no longer acceptable or safe to eat. Highly processed foods tend to have long shelf lives of a year or more. Fresh foods have short shelf lives of a few days to a few weeks. Long shelf life is both good and bad. A long shelf life makes more foods available to more people in hungry parts of the world, for soldiers, or for use in natural disasters. Long shelf life also means the food may be loaded with preservatives!

Food Claims

A food claim is a statement made by the food producer and printed on the product label to inform consumers of the food's main benefit. For example, "Good source of fiber" or "Gluten-free" are food claims. So is "USDA Organic."

Claims on all products sold in the United States must be true. This truth in advertising applies to cosmetics, laundry detergents, and toilet bowl cleaners, just as it applies to food.

In addition to claiming a food is organic, food producers have invented various other attributes to appeal to consumers. Some of these claims make sense as benefits to the environment, society, or our nutrition, but some other claims seem to be meaningless. Here are the popular food claims made today:

➤ Fair trade certified: Farmers are paid living wages and have safe working conditions, child labor is prohibited, most pesticides are banned, and part of the profit is returned to local community development.

➤ Rainforest Alliance Certified: Farms raising mainly coffee, tea, cocoa, nuts, and fruits follow practices that conserve water and soil and protect wildlife habitat.

➤ Food Alliance Certified: The food producer meets requirements in soil and water conservation, safe and fair working conditions, limited pesticide use, animal welfare practices, and wildlife habitat conservation.

➤ Salmon-Safe certified: The food was produced using methods that protect salmon streams and manage or minimize farm runoff, chemicals added to the environment, water use, and erosion.

➤ Dolphin-Safe certified: This applies to practices used to catch tuna that minimize accidental killing of dolphins and other marine life. Certification requires no encircling of dolphins, no drift gill nets, and no serious injury to dolphins during an entire fishing trip.

➤ Bird Friendly certified: This applies to organic shade-grown coffee, meaning the grower protects the forest canopy, plant diversity, shade coverage of the land, and streamside borders. The goal is to protect bird habitat.

➤ GMO-Free or Non-GMO Project Verified: The foods have been grown without any use of genetically modified organisms (GMOs). A GMO is a plant, animal, or microbe that contains a gene from another organism to give it special favorable characteristics.

➤ Certified Humane Raised and Handled: The food animal producer handles the livestock in a humane manner from birth to slaughter. The farm also maximizes the animals' ability to behave naturally for its species such as grazing, flapping wings, swimming, or exercising.

Some claims that may not mean much are:

➤ Grass-Fed: All cattle eat grass at some point during their raising, so producers may be trying to mislead consumers with this claim. Even grass-fed cattle end up in feedlots sooner or later before going to slaughter.

➤ Cage-Free or Free-Range: This is usually applied to laying chickens. No standards exist for substantiating this, so the cage-free time of the animal's life may be very short. Egg-laying chickens continue to endure some of the worst conditions of any farm-raised animal. The logo stating United Egg Producers Certified does not ensure that the chickens were raised with any more humane treatment than those raised using standard practices.

➤ Cruelty-Free: This implies that the food animals were raised under humane conditions, but this claim is unsubstantiated and subjective. The claim Certified Humane Raised and Handled is better because it is monitored by various animal welfare organizations, including the American Society for the Prevention of Cruelty to Animals (ASPCA).

➤ Environmentally friendly: It means nothing.

➤ Natural: What food isn't?

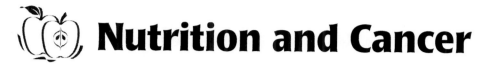

CHAPTER 30

Nutrition and Cancer

In This Chapter

➤ Cancer basics
➤ Cancer-causing constituents of food
➤ Potential cancer-preventing foods

In this chapter I provide an update on the current thinking about nutrition and cancer. This is a broad-reaching subject with no definite conclusions. We know good nutrition can help the body fight many diseases, but nutrients are not a cure for any disease other than specific, known nutrient deficiency diseases. Furthermore, the causes of cancer are numerous and their relationships difficult to determine.

In this chapter, I cover the basics of what we need to know about nutrition and cancer, understanding that the questions far outnumber the answers.

The Nature of Cancer

Scientists consider cancer to be many diseases. It affects different types of cells in the body and occurs in different organs. The causes come from genetics, environment, and lifestyle. The environmental causes can be chemicals, viruses, irradiation, and even tiny particles.

Cancer is an abnormal, rapid, and uncontrolled division of cells. As these cells grow, they form large masses of disorganized cells called tumors. Unlike organs, which are organized and have cells that serve a purpose, tumors do nothing in the body except take up space and draw in nutrients. If a tumor enlarges enough, it presses on nearby organs and can interfere with the healthy organ's normal function. The expansion also often leads to pain.

Tumors are benign or malignant. Benign tumors do not harm normal body functions unless they grow too big and interfere with organs. Malignant tumors (also called malignant neoplasms) cause harm by invading healthy tissue and organs. When malignant tumors spread from their place of origin in the body to other parts of the body, they are said to have metastasized. Metastasis often occurs when some cancer cells break away from the tumor and travel in the bloodstream to a new spot in the body.

Lung cancer is the most common cancer to cause death in the United States. Those who get lung cancer include both smokers and nonsmokers. Breast cancer in women is the next most common cause of death, followed by prostate cancer in men, colon and rectum cancer, leukemia and lymphomas, and those cancers that affect the pancreas, ovary, and liver. Cancer can occur in every tissue of the body.

Cancer-Causing Constituents of Food

Diet may account for up to 40 percent of the cancers diagnosed in the United States. This statement should provide all the impetus you need to examine your dietary habits and correct mistakes that are suspected of being connected to cancer.

While we know some foods have a close connection to increased rates of cancer, other foods may be able to protect against cancer. Let's begin with the foods or nutrients that are possibly carcinogenic (cancer causing):

➤ Total fat: Saturated and polyunsaturated fats are linked with increased cancer incidence. High saturated fat intake is linked with prostate cancer.

➤ Nitrates and nitrites: These preservatives and enhancers of cured meats (bacon, ham, sausages) react with amino acids during cooking to form nitrosamines, known to cause cancer.

➤ Heterocyclic amines: Chemicals that enter meat fat with charcoal broiling, they are linked to stomach and colon cancers.

➤ Aflatoxin contamination of grains: These toxins made by fungi may be present in low amounts on whole grains. Aflatoxin is linked to liver cancer.

➤ Sugar: Sweets loaded with simple carbohydrates cause an insulin surge in the blood. This may aid tumor growth.

➤ Calorie intake: Excessive calorie intake leads to obesity and interferes with normal hormone secretion and function, events that are linked to increased risk of cancer.

Cancer-Protecting Constituents of Food

None of the foods or nutrients listed here are magic bullets in preventing cancer. They certainly cannot cure cancer. But scientists know that the activities of these constituents combat some of the actions of cancer.

The main foods with possible action against cancer are:

➤ Dietary fiber: Linked with decreased colon and rectal cancers, possibly by speeding the movement of material through the digestive tract, carrying carcinogens away.

➤ Vitamin E and vitamin C: Both can prevent nitrosamine production.

➤ Omega-3 fatty acids: It may inhibit some tumor growth.

➤ Linoleic acid (an essential fatty acid): It may inhibit tumor development.

➤ Folate and vitamin A: Both promote normal cell development.

Other food constituents that may have benefits against cancer are vitamin D, calcium, the phytochemicals (flavonoids, indoles, and phenols), and the antioxidants (vitamin E, carotenoids, and selenium).

Foods Against Cancer

Rather than concentrate on particular food constituents to prevent cancer, it's easier to learn the foods that scientists feel may work against cancer.

These foods are:

➤ Soy products: They contain phytic acid, which may bind carcinogens in the digestive tract and thus help carry the chemical out of the body.

➤ Berries: Because of their antioxidant content, they are believed to be beneficial in preventing cancers caused by free radicals from fat metabolism.

➤ Cruciferous vegetables: These are leafy vegetables of the cabbage family (cabbage, cauliflower, kale, collards, and broccoli). They are rich in phytochemicals, which have gained interest as chemicals that protect cells against cancer development.

Other foods that are being recommended for their effects against cancer are: onions, leeks, scallions, garlic, and mushrooms. They contain a variety of phytochemicals thought to prevent tumor development.

CHAPTER 31

Food Allergies and Intolerances

In This Chapter

➤ The main causes of food allergy

➤ How to determine if you have a food allergy

➤ The main causes of food intolerance

➤ Managing allergies and intolerances through diet choice

A previous chapter introduced you to food allergies and food intolerances. In this chapter, the most common causes of these troublesome allergies and intolerances are examined in more detail.

Are food allergies and intolerances increasing? They seem to be as we hear more each day on the evils of gluten, wheat, peanuts, shellfish, and various food additives. Emergency room data indicate that the incidence of serious food allergies is indeed increasing in the U.S. They affect more than 10 million Americans, and a greater percentage of children are affected by these allergies than adults.

Food allergies range from mild to severe or in rare instances can be life-threatening. Therefore, it is important to identify any allergies you might have to certain foods based on the symptoms described earlier in this book. Food intolerances are generally less dangerous to health than allergies. But intolerances are annoying, so we will examine the best ways to avoid both allergens and intolerance-causing substances in food.

The Main Causes of Food Allergy

Food allergy, also called hypersensitivity, is the body's immune system's overreaction to a single constituent in a food. This substance, called an allergen, is almost always made of protein.

The most common foods with allergens are:

➤ Peanuts: Peanut allergies are swift, can be fatal, and are caused by mere trace amounts of peanut residue in food. Three different peanut proteins have been implicated. People known to have this allergy can carry epinephrine injector pens (EpiPens) and inject the epinephrine within 10 minutes of exposure to peanut-containing foods.

➤ Tree nuts: Several different nuts make up this group, mainly walnut, almonds, hazelnut, cashew, pistachio, and Brazil nuts. The proteins in tree nuts are not related to peanut protein. In addition to whole nuts, these nuts show up in a variety of foods, such as pesto, candies and marzipan, cereals, cookies, nut butters, and non-dairy milks. Tree nut allergies range in severity from mild to fatal.

➤ Eggs: This allergy is very common in children but many children outgrow it. The main allergen is albumin protein found in egg white. Any person with severe egg allergy should avoid both egg whites and yolks because some albumin contaminates the yolk when the white and yolk are separated.

➤ Wheat: Common in children up to age three, wheat allergy in adults is often confused with gluten intolerance. Wheat allergy is caused by at least four groups of wheat proteins: albumin, globulin, gliadin, and glutenin (better known as gluten). Albumin and globulin are the biggest culprits in causing allergic reaction. Baked goods are obvious wheat-containing foods, but almost every processed food group has the potential to contain wheat in small amounts. Wheat allergies cause an array of serious symptoms but they are rarely fatal.

➤ Milk: Milk allergy is caused by the protein casein in cow's milk. Many infants develop this allergy and then outgrow it. The allergy's symptoms vary widely from person to person from very mild to very severe. Milk allergy is not the same as lactose intolerance, which is fairly common in adults.

➤ Shellfish: Various muscle proteins in two categories of shellfish cause mild to very severe allergies. The first category contains the crustaceans shrimp, prawn, crab, crayfish, krill, and lobster. The second category contains the mollusks squid, octopus, snails, clams, oysters, and mussels.

➤ Fish: Fish allergies refer to the finned fish (or finfish) rather than shellfish. These allergies also arise when a person is hypersensitive to various fish proteins, some of which have not been identified by scientists. More than 20,000 species of finfish exist and an allergy to one may mean a person will be allergic to additional types. Some of the most popular finfish on menus are tuna, salmon, bass, flounder, catfish, anchovies, halibut, snapper, swordfish, sole, tilapia, trout, mahi mahi, herring, and cod.

➤ Soy: Also called soybean allergy, this is usually mild. This allergy becomes severe in only rare cases. The protein is usually referred to as Soy Protein Isolate and can be present in a variety of foods because soy is used increasingly by food manufacturers as a low-calorie filler and texture enhancer. The easy culprits to spot are soy sauce, soy milk, edamame, tofu, and soy cheese. Soy protein shows up in Asian foods such as miso, tempeh, shoyu, tamari, and natto, and it is also in snack foods, canned soups, baked goods, and many other canned and processed foods.

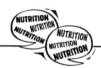

Nutrition Vocabulary

Epinephrine, also called adrenaline, is a hormone released by the adrenal glands when the body reacts to stress. It causes a rapid increase in oxygen supply to the brain, increased glucose flow to the brain and muscles, and a temporary slowing of the digestive tract. When used as a drug, epinephrine counteracts the strong allergic reactions to the proteins in the main allergy foods listed in this chapter.

How to Determine if You Have a Food Allergy

A severe allergic reaction tells you something you may have eaten in a recent meal has triggered your immune system. If the allergic reaction is very uncomfortable for you, but you cannot determine the cause by yourself, seek a certified nutritionist or a doctor to help you find the cause.

The simplest way to identify a food allergy is to write down everything you have eaten. Over time, you should be able to find a connection between a certain food and the allergy. By eliminating the food from your diet, and thus eliminating the allergy symptoms, you can be confident you have identified the exact allergy. A nutritionist can help set up this program so it is done in a logical manner.

Additional tests for food allergies such as a skin test or blood test should be done with the supervision of a doctor. Dietary tests, such as the two listed below, can be performed with the help of either a nutritionist or a doctor. The main tests, from easiest to most labor intensive, are:

➤ Skin test: The doctor injects a small amount of a suspected allergen under the skin and then monitors the injection site. A reaction at the site may take several minutes to a few days to appear.

➤ Blood test: The presence of an antibody called IgE (short for immunoglobulin E) in a person's blood may indicate a specific food allergy. After drawing a blood sample, a medical technician tests the blood against several suspected allergens. If your blood's IgE antibodies react to a specific allergen, you've identified the problem. The results from blood tests usually take several days before producing an answer.

➤ Elimination diet: If you already suspect a certain food allergy, you and your nutritionist (or doctor) can devise a diet lacking that particular food. Stay on this diet for at least two weeks and watch to see if all allergy symptoms clear and do not return.

➤ Food challenge: This test is good for determining the presence of more than one food allergy. In this test a nutritionist or doctor devises a very bland, but nutritionally complete, base diet. Each food suspected of causing allergy is added to the diet one at a time. If no allergy symptoms appear, more foods can be added. As soon as symptoms appear, you can pinpoint the last food that had been added to the diet. This food is likely the cause of your allergy.

Nutrition Morsels

Gluten intolerance is very popular nowadays—almost everyone thinks they have it. Food manufacturers have deftly exploited this fear by producing a near endless array of foods that are "Gluten Free." Even foods that never contained gluten in the first place have jumped on this bandwagon. The symptoms of gluten intolerance vary but usually include gas, abdominal pain, headache, bloating, and occasional diarrhea. Of course, these are also symptoms for many other allergies. Intolerance to gluten can be difficult to confirm because gluten appears in a very wide array of foods so it is not easy to eliminate from the diet.

The Main Causes of Food Intolerance

Unlike food allergies, food intolerances do not involve the immune system. Food intolerances usually require larger amounts of the food than in allergies for symptoms to occur.

Food intolerances have two main causes: (1) lack of a needed enzyme to properly break down the food in the digestive tract, and (2) overreaction by a person's metabolism to an ingredient in food. These overreactions take many forms and may include a change in breathing, blood pressure, or balance. Some food intolerances cause temporary numbness to parts of the body, such as the fingertips, and sweating, vomiting, or headache.

The most common food intolerances are:

➤ Dairy or lactose intolerance: This is caused by a reaction of your normal digestive tract bacteria to the milk sugar lactose. Milk from cows, goats, and sheep can cause this problem.

➤ Wheat intolerance: This problem arises from a reaction to parts of the wheat grain and in some people the grains of rye, barley, and oats. Wheat proteins other than gluten cause this intolerance, marked by bloating, headache, and joint pain. This intolerance differs slightly from celiac disease, which is a reaction to the gliadin protein of wheat, barley, and rye. In celiac disease, a person suffers damage to the lining of the digestive tract. This damage then interferes with absorption of other nutrients.

➤ Yeast intolerance: This problem may be tricky to distinguish from wheat or gluten intolerances because all three are related to baked goods. Yeast also is in fermented foods and alcoholic drinks, beef stock, and salad dressings (in the vinegar). The symptoms are poorly defined and similar to the general symptoms of food intolerance: abdominal pain, gas, diarrhea, weakness, shortness of breath, and rash, hives, or itchy skin.

➤ Histamine intolerance: A person with low levels of the histamine-destroying enzyme diamine oxidase in the gut may experience headache, rash, itching, diarrhea, or vomiting after eating fermented drinks, fermented foods, canned fish, dried fruits, or chocolate.

➤ Alcohol intolerance: This intolerance may be either to alcohol or to the fruit from which the drink was made, such as grapes. It comes from a lack of digestive enzymes needed to break down these foods in the gut. The most common drinks associated with alcohol intolerance are red wine, whiskey, and beer. Symptoms vary but they often mimic those of hay fever: sneezing, runny nose, and coughing.

Some food additives present in tiny amounts can also cause a food intolerance. Because the names of these substances may be far down a list of food ingredients, they are easy to miss and make diagnosis of the illness difficult. In some cases, the offending substance is not listed on the label because it is a natural part of the food, for example, a compound that would be found naturally in bell peppers or pineapples.

Some of the hard-to-find substances that have been linked to food intolerances are:

> ➤ Sulfites
> ➤ Monosodium glutamate (MSG)
> ➤ Food coloring, such as tartrazine
> ➤ Natural amino acids, such as tyrosine
> ➤ Antibiotics added to the feed of food-producing animals
> ➤ Pesticides applied to food crops

Managing Food Allergies and Intolerances

The best approach to managing food allergies and intolerances is to avoid the offending food. Reducing it or eliminating it entirely from the diet is the surest way to avoid symptoms.

Sometimes a person can easily eliminate a food from the diet. For example, a person with a severe allergic reaction to grapefruit should have no trouble planning a grapefruit-free diet for eternity. Other dietary adjustments are more difficult. Wheat, gluten, dairy products, eggs, and yeast are in lots of our foods. If a person suffers allergic reaction or intolerance to more than one of these, planning a safe but nutritionally complete diet can be a challenge.

People with multiple food allergies or intolerances should consult a nutritionist or registered dietician. Work together to find foods that appeal to you but also deliver essential nutrients. A registered dietician can recommend nutrient supplements to ensure a balanced diet.

Some food allergies disappear in time. You may be able to periodically try a small amount of the food every six months or so and watch for the return of symptoms. If you know you have a very severe or life-threatening reaction to a food, do not conduct these experiments by yourself. Consult a professional before devising a test diet or simply avoid the food forever.

Some people overcome mild food allergies by slowly and progressively adding larger amounts of the food back into their diet over time. The body builds up a tolerance to foods that had once caused illness. But this does not always work, so be careful when trying to build resistance to a known food intolerance.

Researchers have come up with a few strategies for allowing allergic people to return some of their favorite foods to their diet. These strategies may not work for everyone, but they are worth investigating further:

➤ Antibody treatment, which allows a person to build up resistance to the food

➤ Vaccines, which similarly build defenses in the body to a specific food allergen

➤ Genetically modified foods that do not contain allergens

The approaches listed here work best for food allergies, which are more serious than food intolerances. Food intolerances are usually solved by keeping the problem food out of your diet, either temporarily or permanently.

Although food allergies and intolerances are annoying or worse, we are lucky to live in a culture with very many food choices. Usually you can find a good substitute for the problem food and return to good health.

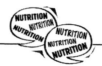

Nutrition Vocabulary

Few things in nutrition cause confusion in the public, as well as some scientists, as the terms "wheat allergy," "gluten intolerance," and "celiac disease." These three conditions are related to very similar food groups and the symptoms are similar too. If you suspect you suffer from one of these, getting a firm handle on which problem you have is useful in adjusting your diet to prevent it.

Wheat allergy is a reaction to wheat proteins by your body's immune system. The reaction is rapid (within 24 hours) and can be severe. Gluten intolerance is a non-allergic reaction (taking hours for symptoms to appear) to the gluten in wheat as well as other grains. (Some allergy researchers believe there is no such thing as a gluten allergy and attribute wheat allergies to other wheat proteins.) Also called non-celiac gluten intolerance, this malady is best solved by eliminating gluten from the diet.

Celiac disease is a pathology, that is, a substance causes damage to a part of the body. In this case, the substance is either of two grain proteins, gliadin or gluten. Celiac disease develops the first time within 24 hours and lifelong damage will occur to the digestive tract unless a person permanently avoids ingesting these two proteins.

CHAPTER 32

Genetically Modified Foods

In This Chapter

- ➤ Introduction to GMOs
- ➤ How to make a GMO
- ➤ Reasons for genetically modifying foods
- ➤ Today's main genetically modified foods
- ➤ Concerns and perspective on GMOs

You have seen the food labels. They assure you a food contains "No GMO Ingredients." What does this assurance mean to your health and even the health of our planet? In this chapter you will learn the basics of GMOs, short for genetically modified organisms. You will be given information to help you decide if GMOs are dangerous, beneficial, or neutral in society and to your personal wellbeing.

A GMO is any plant, animal, or microbe that has been altered by genetic engineering. This chapter will present a handy and simple guide to this technology. It will cover the main plant and animal foods now produced by genetic engineering and will explain how genetically engineered microbes also contribute to food production.

Few subjects in nutrition—or all of biology—are as controversial as genetically modified foods. It's best not to wade into any controversy without mastering the key facts on the subject. We'll begin with an introduction to the science of genetic engineering.

An Introduction to GMOs

Genetic engineering is the mixing of one organism's genetic material, called deoxyribonucleic acid or DNA, with another organism's genetic material. The resulting offspring contain new characteristics they would not normally possess. This is a very powerful tool because every organism's DNA holds all the information needed for survival. Furthermore, DNA holds information from an organism's ancestors and also stores traits to be used by future generations. By altering a DNA molecule, a person can irrevocably change the future course of an organism's progeny.

Genetic engineering has actually been performed since antiquity as people learned to crossbreed plants and animals to develop desirable traits in seedlings or the young, respectively. But crossbreeding takes time. A farmer must wait for generations of crops or livestock before learning which crosses worked best and which did not.

In the 1970s scientists invented laboratory methods that allowed them to snip a piece of DNA from one microbe and insert it into the DNA of another unrelated microbe. Since they were recombining two natural DNA molecules to build a brand new DNA never before seen in nature, the new science was termed "recombinant DNA technology."

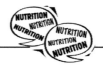

Nutrition Vocabulary

A genetically modified organism, or GMO, is any plant, animal, or microbe that has been created by genetic engineering. Scientists sometimes call the resulting plant or animal a transgenic organism. Transgenic organisms contain genes that were originally present in another organism. If the transgenic organism is a food or food ingredient, it can also be called a genetically modified food.

Recombinant DNA technology gave scientists two big advantages over traditional crossbreeding. First, this technology accelerated the process of developing genetically new offspring. Second, scientists could move very specific pieces of DNA, called genes, to enhance specific traits in the new organism.

Many foods produced in the world today rely on recombinant DNA technology, although we tend to refer to this method of food production as genetic engineering. Genetic engineering has not replaced traditional breeding, which still uses crossbreeding and selective breeding. Both work together. Since the invention of recombinant methods, an entire industry called biotechnology has matured for the purpose of developing drugs and foods through genetic engineering.

Today, genetic engineering plays an important role in global production of crops such as fruits, grains, and vegetables. American consumers have been eating genetically modified foods for about 20 years.

In crop production, farmers use either genetically engineered microbes to increase crop yield or rely on genetic changes to the crop plant itself. Genetic engineering is also increasingly important in food animal production, mainly in fish. When a crop or animal has been developed through the use of genetic engineering, any of the following terms describe the new food: genetically modified food, GMO, or transgenic organism. Some food manufacturers are starting to add the terms GM (for genetically modified) or GE (for genetically engineered) to their food labels.

How to Make a GMO

Biotechnologists can now make a GMO in a matter of weeks or days. All the substances needed for getting DNA out of a cell, cutting out a specific gene, and splicing the gene into new DNA can be purchased from biotech supply companies. A few enzymes, an incubator, and a short list of simple equipment and voilà! A GMO is born.

Here are the basic steps in making a GMO:

1. Grow a flask of a microbe that has a gene for a protein toxic to a certain insect, say a specific caterpillar.

2. Break open the microbe cells and extract all their DNA, which looks like a thick sticky clear liquid.

3. Similarly extract the DNA from a plant such as corn.

4. Use a specific enzyme to cleave the microbe DNA and isolate the caterpillar resistance gene.

5. Break apart the corn DNA in similar fashion and mix it with the microbe's gene. (Actually, thousands of copies of the same microbe gene go into the mix at this step.)

6. Sew together the corn DNA with the new gene using another specialized enzyme.

7. Inject the modified DNA into corn seeds.

8. Grow the new corn plants now containing a gene that makes them resistant to caterpillars.

The above steps show how biotechnologists currently make corn resistant to the advances of a squiggly thing called the European corn borer. The resistance gene comes from common soil bacteria called Bacillus thuringiensis. This microbe is called Bt for short. In addition to enhancing corn, Bt is now used in agriculture to give potatoes, cotton, tobacco, and a variety of garden plants increased resistance to insects. In the early days of Bt's use, farmers put the microbes in water and sprayed the mixture directly on their plants.

Many organic farm supply stores sell Bt as an effective and natural pesticide against mosquitoes and a variety of worms that attack garden vegetables and fruits. At the same time, GMO opponents cite the Bt gene as the starting point on a dangerous path toward genetic manipulation.

Reasons for Genetically Modified Foods

Biotechnology develops crops and food animals for two main purposes: (1) to protect the organism and (2) to give the organism new value. This branch of biotechnology is sometimes called green biotechnology. The following list shows the major reasons for today's genetically modified foods.

> ➤ To protect crops from herbicide damage

> ➤ To protect plants or animals from virus or fungus infection or insect infestation

> ➤ To make crops tolerant to environmental stressors such as drought or flooding

> ➤ To make crops tolerant to changing climate and fish tolerant to warmer water temperatures

> ➤ To increase an organism's production of natural oils, omega-3 fatty acids, or vitamins

> ➤ To make a plant able to produce a drug

> ➤ To develop a plant without certain allergens

> ➤ To make a plant able to produce a pesticide, thus decreasing overall pesticide use

> ➤ To improve a crop's flavor, color, or ripening characteristics, or resistance to bruising during shipping and storage

Opponents of genetically modified foods argue that food manufacturers expose the public to unnatural foods simply to make food production, storage, and shipping cheaper and easier.

These economic benefits of genetic engineering are undeniable, but there are many other reasons for developing genetically modified foods. The reasons touch on today's concerns about environment, pollution, climate change, and global poverty and the hunger it causes.

Nutrition Morsels

Green biotechnology uses genetic engineering to create foods, plants, forests, and animals better suited for today's environment. This branch of science grew out of the dual movements of environmentalism and biotechnology.

As the number of humans on Earth continues to grow past levels the planet can sustain, food, water, land, and even clean air become limited. Green biotechnology cannot solve all these problems but it focuses on the main issues that can be helped through genetic engineering. Scientists in green biotechnology conduct research on the world's main food crops and animals, forests at risk from global warming, and important flowering plants.

Biotechnologists certainly must confront serious concerns on the effect of GMOs in the environment. Green biotechnology, therefore, emphasizes safety mechanisms that must be built into any new GMO it develops.

The global reasons for developing genetically modified foods are:

➤ To maintain crop and seafood yields in areas increasingly affected by climate change; for example, plants with better drought-resistance, flood-resistance, or tolerance of higher temperatures

➤ To reduce chemical pesticide use and the resulting pollution

➤ To increase food yields or combat crop diseases in impoverished regions of the world

➤ To lengthen food storage times as an aid to fighting world hunger

➤ To produce extra nutrients in crops or milk for use in malnourished populations

Many of the above goals have met success, such as drought-resistant plants that demand less water than their traditional cousins. Many of these goals, however, remain on biotechnology's wish list. Progress in genetically modified foods is often slowed by the fierce opposition to these foods, which this chapter will soon cover.

Today's Main Genetically Modified Foods

Most of the existing genetically modified foods have been available for decades in the U.S. and other parts of the world. In Western Europe, by contrast, nations have banned almost all genetically modified foods.

Nutrition Morsels

Climate change and population growth impact global food production in three main ways. First, rising temperatures on land and in the ocean greatly affect the way crops and fish grow. By making plants and animals more resistant to global warming, scientists can help maintain food production for an ever-increasing world population. Second, climate change creates more desert-like conditions and drought in certain regions. Foods that can better withstand these environmental stressors will help overall food production. Finally, climate change will bring higher sea levels and flooding to coastal areas. Some crops, such as rice, are genetically engineered to withstand being underwater for long periods.

Nutrition research was once concerned only with vitamin requirements and good sources of protein. Today, nutrition faces the interconnected dilemmas posed by climate change, overpopulation, and environmental damage.

The foods listed below are the most common genetically modified foods worldwide. This list also shows the main reasons for the genetic altering.

> ➤ Soybeans: Herbicide resistance. Soybean oil also modified to contain increased levels of omega fatty acid

> ➤ Maize (corn): Herbicide resistance

> ➤ Tomatoes: Ripening characteristics

> ➤ Rapeseed (canola) oil: Herbicide resistance

> ➤ Sugar beets: Herbicide resistance

> ➤ Yellow and zucchini squash: Insect and virus resistance

> ➤ Papaya: Virus resistance

> ➤ Alfalfa: Used as a feed for livestock, modified for herbicide resistance

The crops in the above list have been introduced in the U.S. and other parts of the world. Only the genetically modified tomatoes (marketed as FlavrSavr in the 1990s) in the list were not successful. A new generation of genetically modified tomatoes may be on the way. Biotechnologists are developing the following foods and hope to soon see them approved for consumers:

➤ Rice: Insect resistance; higher vitamin A and iron content; increased yield

➤ Wheat: Herbicide resistance

➤ Salmon: Faster growth and bigger size; warm water resistance; disease resistance

➤ Tomatoes: Drought resistance

Many other foods are not genetically modified (called non-GMO foods) but were produced with the help of genetically modified microbes. These microbes produce enzymes that aid cheese making, vitamin content in cow's milk, and certain attributes of eggs used for making egg powder and other egg products. Meat-producing animals often receive hormones that increase weight gain; these hormones are usually made by genetic engineering.

Concerns and Perspective on GMOs

GMOs may have more opponents than allies. Despite the widespread use of genetically modified foods, most countries enforce very strict rules on them. The largest growers of genetically modified foods are the U.S., Canada, Brazil, Argentina, Uruguay, Paraguay, and Australia. China, India, South Africa, Mexico, the Philippines, and parts of Central America and Africa also plant genetically modified crops.

Skepticism abounds on the safety of GMOs, however, in parts of the world. Most Western European countries follow strong edicts by the European Union against genetically modified foods. The United Kingdom, Germany, Italy, France, Austria, Spain, Greece, Portugal, and Luxembourg have partial or almost complete bans on planting, selling, or marketing genetically modified foods.

Even in the countries with widespread use of these foods, opposition to their use is very strong. Some states and cities in the U.S. have tried to ban all GMOs in markets and restaurants. Some opponents have been stridently rigid against all forms of genetic engineering, called these foods "Frankenfoods." (They refer to genetically altered salmon as "Frankenfish.")

The main concerns GMO opponents have relate to both human health and safety for the environment. The arguments against GMOs of any type fall into the following main categories:

➤ Environmental risks of introducing a new gene into a plant or animal

➤ Development of new insect- and microbe-resistant organisms that can take over ecosystems

➤ Release of genetically modified plants and animals into the environment with harm to wild varieties, possibly leading to extinction

➤ Unknown future health risks for humans and wildlife due to these unnatural organisms

Nutrition Morsels

In the U.S. the Food and Drug Administration (FDA) regulates foods from plant sources and their packaging, including foods made through genetic engineering. (This includes animal feeds, but the U.S. Department of Agriculture [USDA] regulates animal-based foods such as meat and milk. The FDA and USDA each regulate different parts of eggs!) Concern from consumers over whether GMOs are "hidden" in our foods have prompted the FDA to publish new guidelines to encourage food manufacturers to tell us on the label if a product contains a genetically modified food.

The FDA has yet to make a decision on labeling food products as "GMO-containing" or "GMO-free." Some states have begun on their own to make rules for labeling foods that contain genetically modified ingredients. Vermont has proposed a labeling law to take effect in 2016. California lawmakers are debating similar regulations. When, or if, these labels appear, they might say "GMO," "GM" for genetically modified, or "GE" for genetically engineered. You already can find many food products that say "GMO-free" on their package. There are no laws against declaring a food as GMO-free.

Opponents of GMOs also question whether genetic manipulation truly helps crop yields or makes plants and animals sufficiently resistant to pests. The public has learned through experience that hormones and antibiotics fed to meat- and milk-producing animals have turned up in the environment and cause harm there. Antibiotics in animal feed may be a major cause of antibiotic resistance now complicating human healthcare.

Many factors unrelated to agriculture lead to worldwide hunger. For example, politics and poverty are intertwined in many parts of the world and cannot be solved by green biotechnology. Likewise, green biotechnology cannot by itself undo environmental decay and climate change.

Foods today are mass-produced and travel long distances from farm to table. You are right to be concerned about the quality of many of the foods you buy. Vitamins and other nutrients can deplete over time in some foods, while a long list of chemical ingredients on the package may make you pause. For that reason, many people simply do not want genetically modified ingredients in their food as a precaution against possible health risks.

Keep genetically modified foods in perspective. They have not yet been proven to be safe. On the other hand, we have been eating them for decades and they give no indication of being unsafe. Time will tell whether the potential benefits outweigh any possible risks.

APPENDIX A

Glossary

acute disease: A disease with a sudden onset, severe symptoms, and a rapid recovery

aerobic: Any biological process that uses oxygen in its chemical reactions; for example, respiration

allergen: A foreign substance, usually a protein, that causes an exaggerated response by the body

antioxidants: Chemicals that neutralize the harmful chemical by-products of oxygen reactions called free radicals

bacteria: Single-celled microscopic organisms that perform almost every biological reaction on Earth; normal inhabitants of the environment and the intestines

ben oil: Extract from the horseradish tree family that contains behenic acid and several essential fatty acids

bioaccumulation: The increased concentration of certain chemicals moving up a food chain

bioavailability: The extent to which a nutrient is absorbed by the intestines and thus available for use by the body

bulimia: An eating disorder characterized by an insatiable appetite, overeating, binge eating, and often self-induced vomiting

carbon footprint: A person's or population's effect on the environment determined by the amount of resources used and the amount of wastes produced

cartilage: Specialized dense connective tissue that withstands pressure and tension and strengthens parts of the body

centrifugation: Spinning a liquid at very high revolution speeds to separate different constituents of varying densities

chlorophyll: A light-capturing pigment contained in photosynthetic plants, algae, and some bacteria

chronic disease: A disease with a gradual onset, long-term duration, and a slow recovery

cilia: Tiny hairlike appendages on the surface of some body cells

compound: A group of atoms of different chemical elements that combine in specific proportion

converted rice: Brown rice that has been heated to give it the texture and appearance of white rice but with the nutrients of the whole grain

cytochrome: A biological pigment that performs specific functions in cells, such as the transfer of electrons in respiration or the transport of oxygen in blood

dermatitis: Inflammation of the skin

diverticulitis: Inflammation of the diverticula, pouches that develop along the large intestine

DNA: Deoxyribonucleic acid, this nucleic acid serves as the storage compound of hereditary information and controls the production of new cell proteins

electron: The smallest part of an atom; it is a particle carrying a single negative charge

emulsify: To suspend fat in water by dispersing the fat into tiny individual droplets

fatty acid: The major part of most lipids, it is a chain of carbons carrying hydrogen atoms

ferment: To derive energy from an organic compound without using oxygen resulting in a new organic compound, such as alcohol, as the end product

flagella: Flexible tails that help certain biological cells, such as bacteria, protozoa, and sperm cells, move

flavonoids: Also called bioflavonoids, a class of chemicals made by many plants that participate in biological reactions

gene therapy: Treatment of a disease by inserting a new gene into a person's genetic material, DNA, for either replacing a faulty gene or adding a missing gene

genetics: The study of heredity, how genes go from one generation to the next and how individuals get certain traits from their parents

glucocorticoid: A general name for hormones from the cortex region of the adrenal gland

glycogen: A large organic molecule that serves as the body's main storage form of glucose and carbon

glycolipid: Any lipid that has a carbohydrate, usually a sugar, attached to it

glycoprotein: Any protein that has a carbohydrate, usually a sugar, attached to it

growth hormone: A protein hormone that stimulates animal growth, especially in bones

hormone: A substance made by an organism's body in one location, then secreted to work in another location of the body

interstitial fluid: Body fluid located between organs and outside tissues and cells

irritable bowel syndrome: A generalized condition of the large intestine characterized by gas, inflammation, pain, and irregular stools

kidney stones: Formations of solid or crystalline pebbles that develop in the kidney and can block urine flow

lecithin: A phosphorus-containing lipid (phospholipid) that serves as a constituent of cell membranes, helps emulsify fats in the intestines, and is added to foods as an emulsifier

lipid: A compound made of carbon and hydrogen, little oxygen, and sometimes other elements and is insoluble in water and helps in membrane and nerve function, among other functions, in the body

lymph: A clear fluid that travels through the body in vessels that make up the lymphatic system; helps carry fats through the body and participates in immune function

macrobiotic: A type of diet that emphasizes whole grains, fish, and minimal processed foods

macromolecule: Any large molecule, such as proteins, fibers, nucleic acids, complex lipids, and some vitamins

macular degeneration: Loss of pigments in the eye's retina leading to impaired vision

marbling: Streaks of fat without muscle that adds flavor and tenderness to steaks and some other meats

membrane: Any fragile divider between two fluids or the covering of cells and tissues; membranes protect cells by preventing certain substances from crossing from one side to the other

metabolic rate: The rate by which the body uses energy

mineral: An inorganic element used by the body to help specific chemical reactions and to form body structures, such as teeth and bone

molecule: An electrically neutral combination of atoms held together as a unit and has distinct chemical properties, such as a molecule of water (hydrogen-oxygen-hydrogen, or H_2O)

mucosa: Specialized tissue layer that lines hollow organs and the body cavities that are exposed to the environment, such as the eyes, mouth, digestive tract, nasal passages, and genitourinary tract

nucleic acid: Large biological chemicals involved in genetic transfer of information from parents to offspring; deoxyribonucleic acid (DNA) and ribonucleic acid (RNA)

nutrient: A chemical in food that contributes to health by providing energy and the elements needed for building new cells, tissues, organs, and other body constituents, and running the body's chemical reactions

organ meats: Non-muscle meat products such as liver, kidneys, heart, and brain

pathogen: A disease-causing microbe or parasite

peroxide: An oxygen-containing chemical that is often a by-product of normal oxygen metabolism

phosphate: A phosphorus and oxygen-containing chemical group (PO_4) that attaches to other chemicals and plays a role in biological energy metabolism

polyp: An outgrowth or tumor, usually that bleeds, growing in organs with a plentiful supply of blood vessels, such as the colon, rectum, uterus, or nose

polypeptide: A string of many amino acids, like a protein, but without the function of a fully formed protein

polysaccharide: A string of sugars of the same type (starch) or different types (hemicellulose)

prolactin: A protein hormone that stimulates milk production in mammals

protozoa: Single-celled microbes of aqueous environments with more complex internal structures than bacteria; normal inhabitants of the environment and the intestines

R group: A chemical group that is always attached to the main frame of an amino acid and gives each amino acid a unique structure

ribosome: A tiny intracellular structure that numbers in the hundreds to thousands in cells and serves as the site of protein production

semipermeable membrane: A membrane that keeps specific substances from crossing from one side to the opposite side but allows other specific substances to cross freely

skeletal muscle: Muscle fibers that are attached to the body's skeleton and are used primarily for movement

solvent: Any liquid that dissolves a chemical substance

sphincter: A circular muscle that when constricted can prevent the flow of substances from one organ (or section of an organ) to the next

stroke: A sudden loss of nervous system function due to an injury to the blood vessels of the brain

tallow: Fat derived from suet, which is the hard fat of the loins of cattle and sheep

tissue: Collection of cells adapted to perform a specific function in cooperation with each other, such as brain tissue, muscle tissue, or blood

triglyceride: A major form of lipid made from a glycerol backbone carrying three fatty acids on each glycerol carbon

vegan: A person who eats only plant foods or a diet based on only plant foods

INDEX

ABOUT THE AUTHOR

Anne Maczulak, PhD, is the author of over ten books on biology and ecology including Allies and Enemies: How the World Depends on Bacteria, and The Five-Second Rule and Other Myths about Germs. Anne has contributed to articles on germophobia, the fear of germs, in Psychology Today and has been a regular guest on television and radio, speaking to viewers about the good and bad microbes that lurk in households. As a regular guest expert on Martha Stewart Living Radio (Sirius/XM Radio), Anne answers callers' questions on disinfectants, infection, food-borne germs, and other topics in germ-fighting. Anne has spoken to professional hygiene organizations on the best ways to disinfect surfaces. She consults for drug and biotechnology companies as well as laboratories that test new antimicrobial products.

Anne's audiences benefit from her ability to transform complex subjects into easy-to-understand lessons. And yet, reading Anne's books on biology, ecology, and microbiology never feels like reading a textbook. Anne always relates technical topics to the "big picture" and writes for non-scientists.

As a PhD in nutrition with a specialty in microbiology, Anne studied the relationship between intestinal microbes and how humans and other animals use nutrients. During her career in industry, Anne studied microbes of the skin and scalp, the bacteria in drinking water, and microbes of the environment that produce useful cold-tolerant enzymes.